Physiotherapy: Foundations for Practice

Series Editors: Janet H. Carr & Roberta B. Shepherd

Key Issues in Cardiorespiratory Physiotherapy

Editors:
Elizabeth Ellis
Jennifer Alison

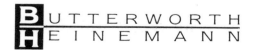

Butterworth-Heinemann Ltd
Linacre House, Jordan Hill, Oxford OX2 8DP

 PART OF REED INTERNATIONAL BOOKS

OXFORD   LONDON   BOSTON
MUNICH   NEW DELHI   SINGAPORE   SYDNEY
TOKYO   TORONTO   WELLINGTON

First published 1992

British Library Cataloguing in Publication Data
Key Issues in Cardiorespiratory
  Physiotherapy. – (Physiotherapy:
Foundations for Practice Series)
  1. Alison, Jennifer   II. Ellis, Elizabeth
  III. Series
  616.1

ISBN 0 7506 0173 6   1824213 8

Library of Congress Cataloguing in Publication Data
Key issues in cardiorespiratory physiotherapy/editors, Elizabeth
  Ellis, Jennifer Alison.
  p.   cm. – (Physiotherapy)
  Includes bibliographical references and index.
  ISBN 0 7506 0173 6
  1. Cardiopulmonary system – Diseases – Physical therapy.   I. Ellis,
  Elizabeth MSc.   II. Alison, Jennifer, MSc.   III. Series:
  Physiotherapy (Oxford, England)
  [DNLM: 1. Cardiovascular Diseases – rehabilitation.   2. Physical
  Therapy.   3. Respiration Disorders – rehabilitation.   WF 145 K44]
  RC702.K49   1992
  616.2'00462–dc20
  DNLM/DLC
  for Library of Congress
                                                    91–47918
                                                    CIP

Photoset, printed and bound in Great Britain by
Redwood Press Ltd, Melksham, Wiltshire

Physiotherapy: Foundations for Practice

Key Issues in Cardiorespiratory Physiotherapy

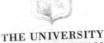

Contents

List of Contributors   vii

Series Editors   ix

Series Editors' Preface   xi

Preface   xiii

Acknowledgements   xv

1   Clinical decision-making in cardiorespiratory physiotherapy   1
    Elizabeth Ellis
2   Assessment of the respiratory system   5
    Colleen Kigin
3   Pulmonary function tests: performance and interpretation   24
    Jennifer Alison
4   Chest radiology   56
    Margaret Stewart
5   Ventilatory dysfunction   80
    Amanda Thomas and Elizabeth Ellis
6   Mucociliary clearance   105
    Jennifer Pryor
7   Pulmonary limitations to exercise performance   131
    Jennifer Alison and Elizabeth Ellis
8   Exercise rehabilitation in cardiac disease   158
    Kathy Henderson

APPENDICES
A   Clinical reasoning: case studies   170
    Elizabeth Ellis
B   Positioning   180
    Jennifer Alison

Index   189

Contributors

Jennifer Alison, DipPhty, MSc (Lond.)
Lecturer, School of Physiotherapy,
Faculty of Health Sciences, Cumberland College, The University of Sydney,
Australia.

Elizabeth Ellis, Grad DipPhty, MSc (Boston), PhD
Senior Lecturer, School of Physiotherapy, Faculty of Health Sciences,
Cumberland College, The University of Sydney, Australia.

Kathy Henderson, BAppSc (Phty), Grad Dip Sports Phty, MAppSc (Hth Sc)
School of Physiotherapy, Curtin University, Shenton Park, Western
Australia.

Colleen Kigin, BS, MS
Director, Chest Physical Therapy, COX 3, Massachusetts General Hospital,
Boston, USA.

Jennifer Pryor, MSc, FNZP
Physiotherapy Department, Royal Brompton National Heart and Lung
Hospital, London, England.

Margaret Stewart, MB, BS(Syd), FRACR, DDR
Department of Radiology, Royal Prince Alfred Hospital, Sydney, Australia.

Amanda Thomas, BAppSc(Phty)
School of Physiotherapy, Faculty of Health Sciences, Cumberland College,
The University of Sydney, Australia.

Series Editors

JH Carr, DipPhty, MEd, EdD, FACP
RB Shepherd, DipPhty, MEd, EdD, FACP

The series editors are associate professors in the School of Physiotherapy, Faculty of Health Sciences, The University of Sydney, Australia and have collaborated on several books and articles. They are developing, based on movement-related research, a theoretical framework for the rehabilitation of individuals with movement disability and have illustrated its use in the rehabilitation of individuals following stroke.[1,2] As a result of this theoretical work, they have been invited to lecture and present papers both overseas and in Australia. Their individual research interests lie in investigating normal and disabled performance of everyday motor actions.

1. Carr J.H., Shepherd R.B. (1987). *A Motor Relearning Program for Stroke*, 2nd edn., Oxford: Butterworth-Heinemann.
2. Carr J.H., Shepherd R.B. eds. (1987). *Movement Science. Foundations for Physical Therapy in Rehabilitation*. Rockville, Md.: Aspen.

Series Editors' Preface

Modern physiotherapy is in the process of considerable change. Physio-therapists are increasingly turning away from a therapeutic function based principally on a medical diagnosis, to an analytic, diagnostic[1] and thera-peutic function, based on biological science, behavioural science and bio-mechanics, in which the medical diagnosis is just one of many sources of information relevant to clinical practice. From its original development as an extension of medical practice (hence the term 'paramedical'), physiotherapy is emerging as an independent applied science.

We have proposed elsewhere[2,3] that the broad area of movement science, which encompasses those parts of the biological and behavioural sciences and biomechanics that are related to human movement, should form the basis from which rehabilitation strategies are developed and tested. This view, we believe, will take physiotherapy into the next century as a health science with its own distinct clinical expertise, equipped also to contribute significantly, through experimental investigation, to the understanding of human function.

The role of the modern clinical physiotherapist in the identification and analysis of problems, therapeutic applications and the improvement of functional motor performance must, therefore, increasingly depend upon four factors: 1) keeping up to date with progress in the relevant behavioural and biological sciences, and biomechanics; 2) developing the judgement to see and understand what is relevant to clinical practice in such theoretical and data-based information; 3) devising analytic and intervention strategies from this material; and 4) testing whether or not these strategies lead to improvement in human performance, whether it be physiological or be-havioural. The role of the academic and research physiotherapist must increasingly be to investigate clinical observations as part of enriching the data-base on human behaviour.

The purpose of this series of books is to illustrate three processes critical to clinical practice: the deduction of clinical implications from theoretical and data-based material; the development of intervention and measure-ment strategies for clinical practice; and the testing of outcome. With this in mind, each volume in the series will include chapters designed to incor-porate up-to-date theoretical and data-based information together with illustrations of the use of this information in the identification and analysis of specific clinical problems and in the development and testing of intervention strategies. It should be noted that the individual books are designed to illustrate the *process* out of which clinical practice emerges. Each book will provide, therefore, a selection rather than a complete coverage of what may be considered relevant material.

The series is designed principally for undergraduate physiotherapy students in order to help them acquire the mental skills necessary for becoming a clinician and for qualified physiotherapy clinicians who wish to update their knowledge. Post-graduate research students will find questions raised that should stimulate a vigorous search for answers.

JH Carr, RB Shepherd
Series Editors

1. Sahrmann S. (1988). *Diagnoses by physical therapists. Applications to trunk imbalance.* Paper presented at the Annual Conference of the Australian Physiotherapy Association, Canberra.
2. Carr J.H., Shepherd R.B. (1987). *A Motor Relearning Programme for Stroke.* 2nd edn, Oxford: Butterworth-Heinemann.
3. Carr J.B., Shepherd R.B., eds. (1987). *Movement Science Foundations for Physical Therapy in Rehabilitation.* Rockville, Md.: Aspen.

Preface

This book has been designed to provide students and educators with a conceptual framework for studying the area of cardiorespiratory physiotherapy. This framework can be used by students of physiotherapy to build their understanding of the interaction between normal physiology, pathology and therapeutic intervention in the area of cardiorespiratory physiotherapy. In addition, it can help students to develop therapeutic strategies through their understanding of relevant scientific material. During subsequent professional development, this framework can be extended as knowledge is drawn from a wide variety of sources. Many of the ideas in this book have been developed over a long period of time and are offered in the hope that they may encourage the same sort of pleasure and satisfaction from working and teaching in the area of cardiac and respiratory physiotherapy for others as we have found ourselves.

An integral part of the conceptual framework is the application of clinical reasoning to the process of decision-making in cardiorespiratory physiotherapy. The ability to make a sound clinical decision as an independent practitioner and to be responsible for that decision is what distinguishes professional training from technical training. Clinical decision-making is an integral part of all areas of physiotherapy and is vitally important when the therapist is working with critically ill people whose condition can change rapidly.

The book is designed to provide examples of commonly occurring clinical conditions and not to be an exhaustive reference on pathology, medicine and therapeutic regimes. We hope the book will encourage readers to seek out relevant material from other sources which will enrich their understanding and, ultimately, their clinical practice. When the word 'patient' is used within the text, it is not intended to imply that the person who is the recipient of the intervention needs to adopt a passive or dependent role. In fact it has been our intention to point out ways in which people who need intervention can manage their own condition when appropriate.

The chapters of this book can be used for different educational purposes. Some chapters should be used as a reference, such as Chapter 3, Pulmonary Function Tests. Others tell a more complete story and demonstrate how the integration of knowledge from a number of fields such as applied anatomy, pathophysiology and respiratory, cardiac and muscle physiology can provide depth to the analysis of individual clinical problems. One such chapter is Chapter 7 which deals with the Pulmonary Limitations to Exercise Performance. Others can be used as a spring board for discussion. For example, Appendix A provides clinical examples which could be used in the undergraduate classroom.

Elizabeth Ellis
Jennifer Alison

Acknowledgements

The editors wish to thank the series editors, Janet Carr and Roberta Shepherd, for their support, patience and editorial assistance throughout the development of this book. We would also like to express our appreciation to Sandra Anderson, Peter Bye, Iven Young and Peter Donnelly for their helpful comments, and Ann Tully and Marita Lennon for their advice from a clinical perspective. Many of the illustrations were skilfully penned by Des Lauff and Denise Nixon.

Chapter 1

Clinical Decision-making in Cardiorespiratory Physiotherapy

ELIZABETH ELLIS

CLINICAL DECISION-MAKING

The process of clinical decision-making is considered circular since the outcome of intervention leads on to further assessment and planning as illustrated in Figure 1.1. The successful outcome will eventually lead to termination of treatment or referral to other practitioners.

Assessment

The assessment phase is a data-gathering phase. The methods used to collect information about the patient are described in detail in Chapters 2, 3 and 4. Included in the assessment phase are the case history notes, discussion with the patient on the history of the present condition and any relevant past history, observation of any signs or symptoms, palpation and auscultation of the thorax, and the interpretation of any relevant tests of lung or cardiac function and exercise tolerance.

Sometimes only part of the assessment can be performed if, for example, the person is unconscious. In this case, the therapist is more dependent on the physical examination and objective tests as the main components of

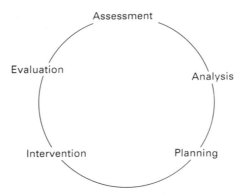

Figure 1.1   Circular model.

assessment. At other times, for example when healthy lifestyle changes are being considered, discussion with the patient is a more important part of the assessment. Information should be carefully recorded so that it can be used in the analysis phase.

Analysis

The analysis phase involves the interpretation and integration of the information gathered from all the above sources. The goal of this phase is to identify those aspects of the person's condition which will respond to physiotherapy intervention. When these aspects or components are identified, an order of priority needs to be established which takes into consideration the effect that intervention will have on the patient's overall condition. The quality of the analysis depends on the ability of the therapist to identify the relevant signs and symptoms, the skill and experience the therapist has developed in working with people and the extent of the therapist's background knowledge.

Planning

The purpose of planning is to establish the goals of intervention and to select the means for achieving these goals. When planning intervention, the relative benefits and risks offered by that intervention should be considered and precautions should be taken to minimize any risks. For example, additional monitoring such as oximetry can be useful when using certain techniques such as suctioning in hypoxaemic patients. It may be necessary to plan carefully the sequence of techniques so that optimal benefit of intervention is achieved.

Intervention

Intervention involves implementing strategies and techniques identified in the planning stage. The therapist must be prepared to be flexible and adapt the intervention depending on the response of the individual. For example, after major thoracic surgery individuals will respond very differently to postoperative pain. Some may feel the pain severely and yet will insist on participating actively in the postoperative procedures. Others will not be able to move and resist strongly any suggestion to do so. It is often the latter who are most likely to develop complications. The therapist must be prepared to use persuasion to prevent a longer recovery.

Evaluation

Evaluation is necessary to assess the effectiveness of intervention. It provides an opportunity to validate the assumptions which may have been made in the analysis phase of the decision-making process. Often goals are refined on the basis of the outcome of the initial intervention.

When assessing the effectiveness of intervention, the therapist should use appropriate measurements for the expected outcome. For example, if a therapist is working with a postoperative patient with lower lobe atelectasis and the goal of intervention is to improve the ventilation to the lower lobe, it would be inappropriate to gauge improvement before and after treatment using measurements of forced vital capacity with spirometry. However, although spirometry provides an objective measure of the maximal volume of air that a person can breathe out, it tells us nothing about the distribution of that air within the lungs. It is also an effort-dependent test which is affected by pain. Therefore, while it is an advantage to have an objective measure, the need for objectivity should not override the need for validity. In this case, auscultation may provide a more relevant measure of improvement in air entry to the atelectatic area even though it is a less objective measure. In addition, regular chest X-rays provide an indication of the longer term progress of the intervention.

One problem for the therapist is that the heart and lungs are internal organs which make direct measurements of the effects of intervention difficult unless invasive techniques are used. To overcome this limitation, information combined from various assessment procedures such as auscultation, changes in the chest X-ray, and changes in arterial blood gases, may be necessary to provide evidence of changes after intervention. If evaluation indicates that the goals of the intervention have been achieved then the therapy may be progressed or terminated as appropriate.

Recommendations

Conclusions made after evaluation of the effectiveness of the intervention can be used in the form of recommendations for ongoing intervention. If the goals were achieved then the treatment can be progressed. If the goals are not achieved or an unsatisfactory rate of progress occurs, then the therapist repeats the decision-making process until a satisfactory outcome is achieved. A more thorough assessment may be needed, or more information may have become available that allows a clearer picture of the patient's condition. It may be that the method of treatment needs to be carried out more vigorously, or more frequently, or integrated with other therapies, such as pain relief or bronchodilators, to be effective. Recommendations can be made for the frequency and intensity of the intervention and to the expected rate of progression and likely outcome. Consideration can be given at this stage to the long-term management and prevention of future episodes or complications. Alternatively, if there is a limit to the effectiveness of physiotherapy intervention, the person could be referred to other health or welfare professionals as required.

SUMMARY

Clinical decision-making is enhanced by using a logical process of assessment, analysis, planning, intervention, evaluation and recommendations. Constant reference to this process ensures that therapy is appropriate and responsive to the changing clinical status of the patient. A physiotherapist's skills are not limited to the ability to make wise clinical decisions. The decision-making process needs to be complemented by clinical skills, effective communication and the ability to analyse and resolve situations where there is ethical conflict. In addition, physiotherapists need to be able to organize their time and their work load in order of priority and record their decisions, intervention, outcome and recommendations so that the records can be interpreted accurately at a later date or by another person.

FURTHER READING

Barrows H.S., Feltovich P.J. (1987). The clinical reasoning process. *Medical Education*, **21**, 86–91.

Magistro C.M. (1989). Clinical decision making in physical therapy: A practitioner's perspective. *Phys. Ther.*, **69**, 525–532.

Payton O.D. (1985). Clinical reasoning process in physical therapy. *Phys. Ther.*, **65**, 924–928.

Watts N.T. (1989) Clinical decision analysis. *Phys. Ther.*, **69**, 569–576.

Woolf S.L. (1985). *Clinical Decision Making in Physical Therapy*. New York: F.A. Davis.

Chapter 2

Assessment of the Respiratory System

COLLEEN KIGIN

INTRODUCTION

Assessment of the respiratory system with the eyes, hands and ears has been done for centuries, and today these methods of gathering information are augmented by modern technology which is used to assist in the analysis and interpretation of the clinical signs and symptoms. This chapter will outline the basic techniques of respiratory assessment, including assessment of various lung pathologies. The value and accuracy of assessment rely heavily on the skill, expertise, and manner of the clinician. The good clinician will refrain from making a quick or even predetermined judgement of the person's problems, but rather wait until as much information is gathered as is necessary for an adequate analysis of the person's condition. A thorough, systematic approach can prevent the clinician from being drawn towards an obvious defect or problem, without a more complete assessment which may provide information as to why or how a condition occurred. This is in contrast to looking only at obvious symptomatology; and perhaps directing care to a symptom without recognizing the precipitating factor or cause.

The clinician should prepare for the assessment by having an organized, predesigned plan which can be adapted for individual needs and circumstances. The basic elements to be included are:

I Clinical History
    a   from the medical records
    b   from personal interview
II Physical Assessment
    a   observation
    b   palpation
    c   percussion
    d   auscultation
    e   functional capacity

The clinician should not only approach the patient with a predetermined outline of the assessment, but also have the necessary equipment. This may be as basic as a stethoscope and clock with a second hand. If the person is ambulatory, a hallway in which to walk may also be useful for assessing functional capacity.

CLINICAL HISTORY

Medical Records

The information gained from a review of the patient's complete medical record, including the past history, can be invaluable in the subsequent assessment of the individual. One of the pitfalls of reviewing a record is the preconception that it requires hours of undivided attention. The goal is to learn to scan a history quickly, pulling out major factors or data pertinent to the present assessment. The clinician rarely has an hour for chart review prior to beginning the physical assessment. The skilled clinician prepares a mental or written outline of information that could prove valuable in the subsequent assessment and treatment plan. These include (building on each other):

(i) Childhood history of pulmonary disease or problems, including frequent colds or pneumonia, frequent bouts of bronchitis, asthma or airway sensitivity, allergies, tuberculosis, croup, epiglottitis, or cystic fibrosis; any surgical procedure, with particular attention to cardiac, thoracic, or upper abdominal procedures and subsequent pulmonary problems.

(ii) Adolescent or adult history of pulmonary diseases; history of smoking; shortness of breath with activity; history of surgical procedures, with special attention to thoracic or upper abdominal procedures and subsequent pulmonary problems; environmental exposure or sensitivity to substances such as animals, fabrics, dust, food, cold, heat; exposure to pollutants including coal dust and asbestos. The length of smoking and number of cigarettes smoked per day should be recorded; and are often noted in pack/year history, for example: 2 packs of cigarettes/day for a period of 20 years = 40 pack/year history.

(iii) Occupation and the impact of occupation on disease.

(iv) Functional capacity and the potential impact of disease on functional capacity.

(v) Present complaint, signs and symptoms including cough, dyspnoea, sputum production, fever, chest pain.

(vi) Diagnostic evaluative data including pulmonary function tests, X-rays, oxygen saturation levels, arterial blood gases, cardiac or pulmonary stress tests.

(vii) Treatment plan by other health professionals including prescribed drug therapy, oxygen therapy and mechanical ventilatory support.

Personal Interview

The ability to elicit additional information efficiently and skilfully from the patient can provide a basis for suspected problems, which can then be verified or dismissed with the physical examination. The clinician who can be efficient yet calm and open to the patient can reap the greatest return. The following specific issues should be considered.

The patient will often provide only sketchy information, or broad categories of problems, waiting for you to acknowledge that he/she can feel free to provide more detail in various areas. The patient will be relying on cues from the therapist to continue or to be more detailed.

The patient who is short of breath or dyspnoeic cannot respond in long sentences without further discomfort. Try to structure the cues so that you obtain the information you desire, but allow the person to answer with a few words—even a 'yes' or 'no'.

Some questions may need to be open-ended, some very structured. Usually, an open-ended question or one that covers a general category can lead to more detailed information in a specific area. Some questions may need to be worded very carefully, for example, 'Are you a smoker?' will often draw a negative response in the hospital environment. 'Have you ever smoked cigarettes?' usually gets more accurate information, especially when followed up by 'If so, how many and for how long?'

Elements to be covered in a patient interview (including verification or clarification of patient record) should include:

1 General health history, with emphasis on pulmonary problems
   (a) Disease processes such as pneumonia, asthma, frequent colds or allergies.
   (b) Health habits such as exercise and smoking.
2 Environmental factors
   (a) Job history.
   (b) Exposure to pollutants (including other smokers in the household or frequented places).
3 Present complaint—Note should be taken of the behaviour of specific signs and symptoms including when they are most severe and what relieves them. Details of the following are particularly important.
   (a) The characteristics of a cough: moist or dry; quality and effectiveness; the time of day or night that it occurs.
   (b) Dyspnoea (difficulty breathing): at rest; on exertion; on lying, flat (orthopnoea); and associated sensations.
   (c) Sputum production: colour, volume, smell, consistency.
   (d) Chest pain: pleuritic, cardiac, gastric or musculoskeletal.
   (e) Precipitating factors and degree of debilitation.

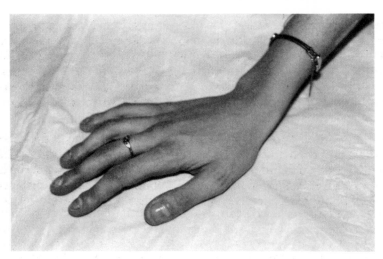

Figure 2.1   The hand of a teenage female with a diagnosis of cystic fibrosis showing clubbed nails. Clubbing may occur with chronic obstructive lung disease, or in younger individuals with lung conditions also resulting in chronic or long term hypoxaemia, such as cystic fibrosis.

PHYSICAL ASSESSMENT

Assessment is routinely divided into four major categories, which include observation, palpation, percussion and auscultation. A fifth category, functional capacity, will also be discussed.

Observation

The patient's general appearance and comfort can give many clues to the presence and severity of pulmonary dysfunction.

General body evaluation. The general muscle bulk of the person should be examined, including the extremities. Chronic respiratory disease can lead to muscle wasting. The very visible contraction of the accessory muscles in a person with respiratory distress may lead the clinician to assume that these muscles are hypertrophied. However, at autopsy, these muscle groups have been found to be atrophied, with normal adipose tissue loss surrounding them, creating the appearance of hypertrophy or prominence. The person who has experienced long-term debilitation from lung disease also may have marked lower extremity wasting due to inactivity.

The colour of the person's skin can also offer valuable information. Normal or adequate oxygenation results in the skin colour we define as healthy, whether the person has white, brown, or yellow skin. Loss of oxygenation results in a pasty, pale, grey-blue look. This may be easier to observe by looking at the nail beds, or the interior surface of the underlid of the eye. Sometimes the blue colour is not clearly evident, and pressure applied on the nail bed can cause a temporary blanching, and the return of blood flow to the area allows for easier determination of the general colour of the bed. The nail bed itself can change in configuration with prolonged hypoxia, resulting in 'finger clubbing'. The angle of the nail at first becomes less noticeable, and is accentuated as the clubbing progresses (Figure 2.1).

Bony configuration. The normal configuration of the thorax is described in terms of diameters, with the anteroposterior diameter in a ratio of 1:2, in relation to the lateral diameter. That is, the distance or diameter of the chest anterior to posterior should be one half that of the lateral distance or diameter. Abnormalities in the bony configuration are closely related to changes in lung function and include:

1 'Barrel chest'. With many chronic lung diseases where there is hyper-inflation of the lungs, the 1:2 ratio changes dramatically, to a 1:1, or equal ratio. This results in the barrel chest configuration.
2 Kyphoscoliosis is a structural deformity in which the rib cage and vertebral column assume asymmetrical formation, with subsequent impairment or restriction on the lung fields.
3 Pectus carinatum (pigeon or chicken breast) results in the sternum protruding beyond the adjacent ribs, similar to a fowl.

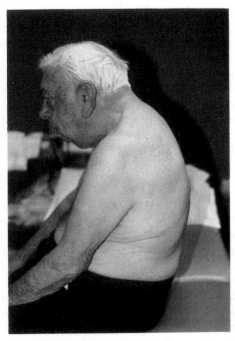

Figure 2.2 *Individual with chronic obstructive lung disease who also has a mild kyphosis, or increased anterior to posterior curvature of the vertebral column.*

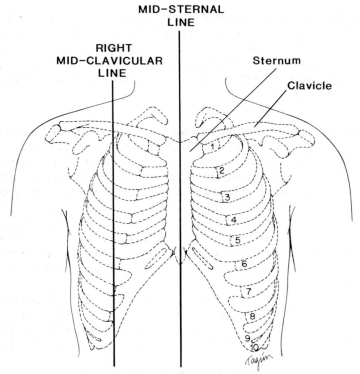

Figure 2.3   Anterior bony landmarks of the thorax. Landmarks used in chest assessment include mid-clavicular line, mid-sternal, and ribs 1–10 anteriorly.

4 Pectus excavatum (funnel chest) results in the sternum being displaced posteriorly beyond the usual configuration. The sternum may be so depressed that it interferes with heart function.

5 Kyphosis is an exaggerated thoracic curvature of the vertebral column with or without an increased anteroposterior diameter of the chest. With ageing this tends to occur naturally; however, the curve may be worse with severe osteoporosis (Figure 2.2).

Bony landmarks. Assessment of the thorax and lungs requires a knowledge of pulmonary anatomy in relation to the bony landmarks. The bony structure of the sternum, the 12 ribs, clavicles, and vertebral column can be used to assist in assessing lung function. General landmarks and terms used in assessing the lung include mid-sternal, mid-clavicular, mid-axillary, scapular line and the vertebral line (Figures 2.3, 2.4, 2.5). The lungs rise 2–4 cm above the inner third of the clavicle, and the bottom border of the lung should be at the 6th rib at the mid-clavicular line, 8th rib on the mid-axillary line, and 10th–12th rib posteriorly (Figures 2.6, 2.7, 2.8). The various lobes are assessed in the position in which they are assumed to be in the thorax. The right upper lobe is usually positioned above the clavicle, down to 4th rib anteriorly (horizontal fissure), and following the medial border of the scapula posteriorly (Figure 2.6). The right middle lobe is positioned between the 4th and 5th anterior rib at the mid-axillary line and down to the 6th rib, laterally to the mid-axillary line (Figure 2.7). The other lobes are delineated in the figures, and should be studied and memorized to proceed with assessment (Figures 2.6, 2.7, 2.8).

Breathing patterns. The normal breathing pattern results in a coordinated, synchronous contraction of the ventilatory muscles and subsequent motion of the thorax. This includes a downward contraction of the diaphragm, resulting in part in a downward excursion of the diaphragm which is palpable but not always easily observed. With the downward contraction of the diaphragm, there is a lateral and upward excursion of the rib cage, providing a 'bucket handle' and 'pump handle' motion (Figures 2.9, 2.10). The abdomen may also protrude slightly on inspiration. Abdominal motion or activity should not be marked or exaggerated during quiet ventilation in the normal adult. However, abdominal motion is very marked in the normal newborn or infant.

The normal respiratory rate should be regular and 12–16 breaths/minute in the normal adult. The infant or small child ventilates at 30 breaths/minute. The flow should be smooth and non-interrupted, and exhalation passive, without noticeable muscle contraction. The inspiratory to expiratory ratio

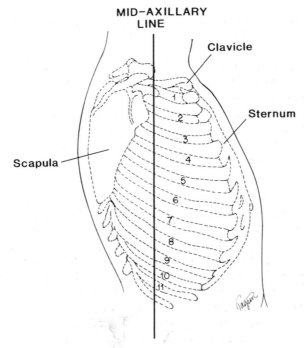

Figure 2.4   Lateral bony landmarks of the thorax including floating ribs 11 and 12 (unmarked).

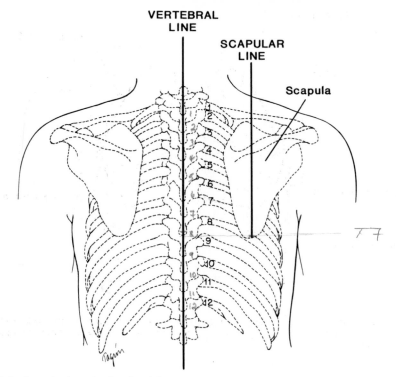

Figure 2.5 Posterior bony landmarks of thorax.

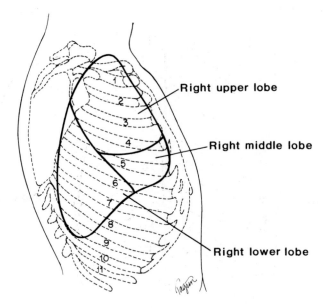

Figure 2.6 Right lung positioned in thorax, with bony landmarks assisting in identifying normal right lung configuration.

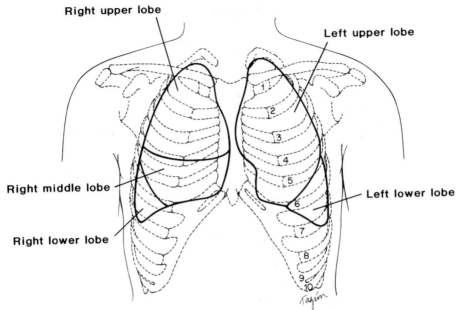

Figure 2.7   Anterior view of the lungs in the thorax in conjunction with bony landmarks. Left upper lobe is divided into apical and left lingula, which matches the general position of the right upper and middle lobes.

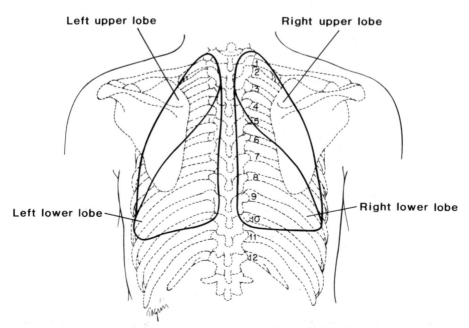

Figure 2.8   Posterior view of the lungs in conjunction with bony landmarks.

should be approximately 1:2, or the time of inspiration one-half that of expiration. Alterations in respiratory rate are referred to as:

1 bradypnoea   slowing of respiration
2 apnoea   temporary absence of breathing
3 tachypnoea   increased rate of respiration
4 hyperpnoea   increased depth of breath
5 hyperventilation   increase in depth and rate
6 periodic ventilation mixture of hyperpnoea and apnoea

Apnoea may occur during sleep, even in normal individuals. Periods of sleep apnoea are not uncommon in the person with chronic obstructive pulmonary disease. Newborn infants may also have sleep apnoea, and may be put on home monitors to help prevent 'cot deaths'. Tachypnoea and hyperpnoea are unusual, marked ventilatory patterns at rest. An increase in rate and depth is a natural response to heavy exertion or exercise, and abnormal with low level activity. The term 'dyspnoea' describes the sensation of shortness of breath, difficulty breathing or breathing that requires effort. The person will complain of a sensation of discomfort, or air hunger. The term refers to the subjective sensation of ventilation but clinical observation may provide clues of increased effort, such as use of accessory muscles. This sensation occurs at rest with severe or acute dysfunction but may occur during exercise with less severe disease. The activities that precipitate the dyspnoea should be noted.

Contraction of accessory muscles of breathing at rest or low levels of activity may be an initial sign of respiratory dysfunction (Figure 2.11). The use of accessory muscles may be normal with high levels of activity. Contraction of the abdominal muscles on exhalation may occur when there is a high expiratory resistance, in conjunction with a prolonged expiratory phase (1:4 ratio) and perhaps use of pursed lips. Abdominal muscles may also be more actively recruited when there is a high respiratory rate or to enhance the length/tension relationship of the diaphragm. Use of abdominal muscles has also been observed at the end of expiration in patients with neuromuscular disease, when rapid relaxation at the beginning of inspiration generates a more negative pressure in the abdomen and enhances the downward movement of the diaphragm.

Costal indrawing is seen with severe respiratory dysfunction when the normal motion of the thorax moving up and out on inspiration is disrupted. The diaphragm, if it is flat enough, may actually be retracting or causing an inward, sinking motion on inspiration. Nasal flaring or a widening of the nares occurs during inspiration with acute distress particularly in infants. This occurs because there are muscles at the nose which are driven in time with the other inspiratory muscles. Purse-lipped breathing occurs when people in respiratory distress breathe out through lips that are drawn together (as a purse string). This has the effect of providing a positive back

9th Rib

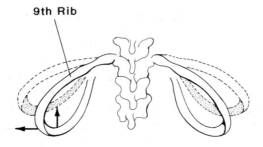

BUCKET HANDLE

Figure 2.9   Bucket handle excursion of ribs is manifested in the lower ribs, where anterior/posterior motion is limited. The bucket handle motion, resulting in the ribs swinging out and up, increases the transverse diameter of the rib cage.

pressure in the airways at the end of expiration which may help to keep the airways open.

Palpation

The palpation of the chest can provide additional information or verification of suspected problems or dysfunction noticed during observation. If a patient has an asymmetrical breathing pattern, palpation of the thorax may result in the ability to differentiate the cause or precipitating factor. The causes of asymmetrical movement could include muscular pain, skeletal or bony pain, or skeletal structural deformity of long standing without pain.

Bony configuration. The ribs should move up and out in a symmetrical pattern during inspiration, and return to the resting position on exhalation. This excursion can be palpated anteriorly around the costal margin and posteriorly by placing the thumbs against the border of the vertebral column

5th Rib

Sternum

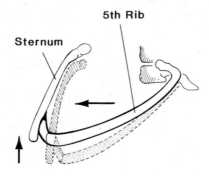

PUMP HANDLE

Figure 2.10   The upper ribs move in a pump handle like motion, increasing the anterior/posterior diameter of the chest.

at the 10th rib, and the fingers spread out over the rib cage. The therapist palpates throughout inspiration and exhalation.

Asymmetrical movement may be due to structural deformity, pain, swelling, or underlying abnormality in the pleural space or lung. An immobile rib cage may be due to muscle paralysis, such as in persons with high level spinal cord injury, or may be due to a constantly hyperinflated position of the thorax or rib cage.

Soft-tissue structures. The assessment should include palpation of any area that is painful, looks swollen, shows atrophy, or has an asymmetrical appearance. In particular, subcutaneous emphysema can be easily detected through palpation, which results in a crackling sensation under the fingers. Subcutaneous emphysema is air in the subcutaneous space, as a result of an incision through the thoracic tissue, or trauma to the chest wall and lung tissue. The presence of air under the skin should be noted, and monitored as the extension or increase of subcutaneous emphysema indicating a continuing leak from the lungs into the tissues.

Palpation of the trachea may identify that it has been displaced due to underlying changes in the mediastinum or lung fields. Space-occupying lesions or tension pneumothorax will push the trachea away from the side of the lesion. A large area of lung collapse will draw the trachea toward the

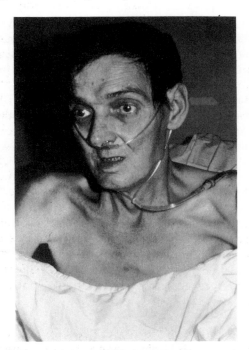

Figure 2.11   A man with chronic obstructive lung disease visibly using accessory muscles to assist in ventilation while at rest. Note the continued use of accessory muscles even with supplemental oxygen being delivered via a nasal cannula.

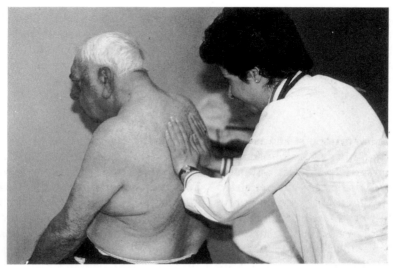

Figure 2.12   The therapist moves her hands down the posterior chest to assess presence and symmetry of fremitus in the posterior lobes while the patient repeats 'ninety-nine'.

lesion. The trachea is easy to palpate below the cricoid rings, and should be midline. Tracheal shift may be confirmed on chest X-ray.

Fremitus. This is a vibration that is transmitted through the bronchopulmonary system as the person speaks. The person is requested to repeat words such as 'ninety-nine', as each lung field is palpated (Figure 2.12). This, as well as other evaluative procedures, should be done symmetrically. The hands should be placed at the apices of each lung, posteriorly, and moved down as the person repeats the words. The vibration will normally decrease as the hands move to the base of each lung. It is particularly important to assess the symmetry of the sensation. A lack of, or decrease in, fremitus can be the result of air in the pleural space (pneumothorax), collapse of the alveoli (atelectasis) or thickening of fluid in the pleura. An increase in fremitus can result when the air spaces are filled with fluid instead of air. This is due to the fact that sound transmits better through a fluid-filled than air-filled medium. Increased fremitus often occurs when a person has a lobar pneumonia. Pleural friction fremitus is felt when the pleural surfaces become inflamed. This results in a pleural friction rub which feels like a grating, and is usually palpated during both phases of ventilation. The pleural surfaces generally have a smooth, uninterrupted surface contact against one another.

Muscle mass. The mass and strength of the general musculature should be included in palpation. This should include the extremities as well as the thorax if the person appears to have atrophy or asymmetrical muscle bulk. The person with chronic obstructive lung disease often has generalized atrophy due to malnutrition associated with the disease. The person with neuromuscular paralysis will have localized muscle atrophy in the area of paralysis. The general appearance of the thorax can lead the examiner to do a general palpation and muscle strength evaluation of the thoracic muscles, including the accessory muscles.

Percussion

Percussion is done by tapping over the surface of the body, which puts the underlying tissues into motion, and results in a vibration or sound. The various sounds can help differentiate an air-filled, fluid-filled, or solid area. The percussion can only penetrate 5–7 cm, but can provide significant information regarding lung function. The proper technique of percussion is crucial to the feedback obtained. The technique can be practised on any surface. The middle finger should be hyperextended (Figure 2.13), and the distal phalanx placed against the skin surface. The other hand is positioned to tap with some force against the extended finger. The first two or three fingers should be tapped through a quick forceful stroke. The tips of the fingers should be at right angles to the extended phalanx. The lightest percussion that will produce a sound should be used.

The differences in tone of the percussive sound differentiates the tissue being percussed. The five basic sounds include: flat, dull, resonant, hyperresonant and tympanic. Percussion should be done in a systematic pattern, just as palpation and auscultation. The percussion should proceed across the lung fields for comparison between lungs, and proceed from the apex to base of each lung. The area percussed should reach down to and below the

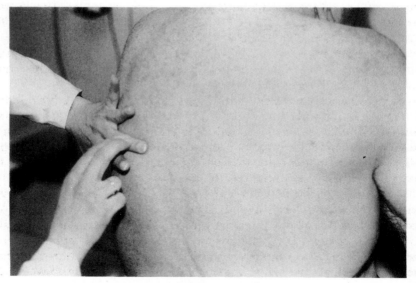

Figure 2.13   The therapist performing percussion on the posterior chest. Percussion would be done from side to side as the therapist moved down the chest wall.

expected position of the diaphragm. The diaphragm will sound dull to percussion, and the percussion tone during full inspiration and at full expiration can help determine the excursion of the diaphragm. Normal progression of sound goes from less resonant in the apices, to more resonant in the bases. However, the muscles and fatty tissue over the thorax can greatly affect the sound expected from person to person.

Hyperresonance will occur normally in children and as a result of hyper-inflated or emphysematous lungs in the adult. Occasionally, there is a hyperresonant sound over a pneumothorax. Dullness will occur when liquid or solid medium is present in the underlying lung. This would be present when there is a consolidation of the lung due to pneumonia, or with a moderate amount of fluid in the pleural space, such as with a pleural effusion. Flatness is a normal sound over the liver or heart, and is heard over the lung fields when a large pleural effusion is present and the underlying lung is collapsed.

Auscultation

Auscultation is the term used to describe the detection of sounds generated within the airways and lung tissue. This evaluative tool has traditionally been listed last, to be used as a final step that has allowed the clinician to pick up cues of expected problems, or underlying disease. However, the clinician may be drawn to use this tool as the sole method of assessment, thereby inadvertently overlooking all the evidence that may be provided by a more thorough physical assessment.

Auscultation may at times be done without the aid of the stethoscope, but the use of the stethoscope allows the sounds to be magnified. The choice of the stethoscope may determine the degree of usefulness of this tool. Two types of stethoscopes include the bell and the diaphragm models. Both are often incorporated into one device. The bell picks up low pitched sounds, such as heart sounds, and the diaphragm picks up the higher pitched tones, such as the breath sounds.

The stethoscope should be placed firmly over the skin, directly against the skin surface. This will eliminate or decrease the interference of sounds from clothing, or those that can occur with light contact of the device against the skin. The patient is instructed to take in a deep breath with the mouth open. Asking the person to breathe through the mouth can eliminate sounds that may be produced in the nose or throat.

Breath sounds should be listened to in a systematic manner, side to side, apices to bases. Each lobe should be listened to, which means that ausculta-tion must take place both anteriorly and posteriorly. Care should be taken not just to listen anteriorly, thereby missing what may be happening in the lower lobes, or only posteriorly, thereby missing the right middle lobe and the lingula segment. Breath sounds are described in a number of ways, all in attempts to further clarify the sound. However, with the terminology so mixed and variant, the clinician may be confused and unable to appreciate the findings of another clinician's evaluation. This chapter will divide the sounds into broad categories, and address the implications of each.

Normal breath sounds. There are two basic sounds heard in the normal lung. They include bronchovesicular and vesicular breath sounds. The bronchovesicular sound is caused by the air flowing in the larger airways and trachea resulting in a louder sound. The sound may be described as tubular, as a result of the large amount of air moving in a large airway. As the therapist listens to the lower or more distal areas of the lung, the sound gradually and normally decreases. This is due to the amount of air per surface area decreasing as the air moves into the smaller airways, or the bronchioles and alveoli. The sounds in this area are termed vesicular.

Abnormal breath sounds. The greatest change in breath sounds between normal and abnormal occurs in the expiratory phase. Consequently, the clinician should pay particular attention to the expiratory phase when listening to the lungs. The abnormal breath sounds may be classified under three general categories:

1 Diminished or absent breath sounds.
2 Added sounds like crackles (crepitations) due to secretion or fluid retention.
3 Added sounds like whistles (wheezes) due to airway obstruction or narrowing.

Diminished or absent breath sounds: These indicate hypoventilation or lack of normal airflow into a lung field which can occur as a result of hypoventilation due to pain, decreased sensorium, or neuromuscular weakness; or it can be due to retained secretions blocking an airway, causing atelectasis or alveolar collapse. The importance of listening to each lung in the apex, mid-lung zone, and base will allow the clinician to ascertain if one lung field is decreased as compared to the other at any one place.

A major difficulty in assessing breath sounds occurs when the sound seems distant or decreased bilaterally, usually at the base of the lung. This can occur post-operatively with general hypoventilation, or due to neuromuscular weakness or paralysis, such as in spinal cord injury. Baseline data available through previous assessments of the patient may be helpful to ascertain if the sounds are decreased as compared with the person's 'normal' condition. The assessment of decreased breath sounds can also be matched to the clinical picture of the patient, including X-ray signs of atelectasis.

Crackles/crepitations/râles: Secretions in the small airways result in a higher pitched sound or a sound like a crackle. As the secretions are cleared, the sound disappears, and is replaced by normal breath sounds. The presence of râles in the periphery of the lung can also indicate atelectasis or alveolar collapse, and this may resolve with simple deep breaths. Râles that do not resolve with either deep breathing or a good cough may be due to intra-alveolar fluid or oedema, and are not usually a result of obstruction or hypoventilation in the airway. Secretions in the large airways result in a large, deep sound that occurs as the air meets the obstruction and moves past it. The sound may clear once the person coughs and clears the secretions. Other terms that may be used are fine râles, medium râles (mucus in bronchioles and small bronchi), and coarse râles (bubbling sounds in larger bronchi).

Whistles/wheezes: The airways transport normal air flow with the resultant normal breath sounds or turbulence transmitted through the stethoscope. However, if the airway is narrowed due to bronchoconstriction, the air is suddenly trying to travel through a narrow opening. As with any narrowed opening, the flow of air can result in a whistle or wheeze. The clinician can grossly differentiate the extent of the airway constriction by the nature of the wheeze. The person who has normal breath sounds at quiet breathing, but a wheeze during forced expiration, has a slight constriction that results in air flow impairment only during a forceful manoeuvre. The person who has more constriction will have expiratory wheezing even during quiet breathing. As the airway narrows further, the wheeze may occur even during inspiration, or at the point of maximal airway distension. This person will be in acute distress due to the high resistance to air flow. The very extreme phase of airway constriction can be a difficult clinical sign, as the breathing may seem remarkably quiet. The clinician must recognize the person who has had significant wheezing and who now has quieter breath sounds and signs of increased respiratory distress, as the airways may be so constricted as to be virtually incapable of transporting air. Localized wheeze can result from a foreign object in the large airway or a growth on the airway, such as a tumour.

Vocal sounds. Normal vocal sounds heard through a stethoscope are not as loud and distinguishable as when directly listening to the person. However, changes in the lung field and pleural spaces can alter the vocal sound heard with a stethoscope and therefore assist in differentiating various conditions. Vocal resonance or bronchophony is the increase in intensity of the voice or spoken word when listening through a stethoscope which results from the presence of fluid in usually air-filled spaces. The fluid, carrying the sound with greater clarity, can result from a pneumonic process with alveoli filled with fluid, or at the edge of a pleural effusion, where the sound is picked up by the fluid bordering the air-filled lung. The term 'bronchophony' is usually used when the resonance is increased in intensity, but the syllables of the spoken word are still not distinguishable. The best way to describe these changes is to state that the sound of the voice suddenly jumps out at you through the stethoscope, in an area where the sound should be decreased. Whispered pectoriloquy occurs when the syllables are understandable, and the sounds jump out at you through the stethoscope even as the person is whispering. This indicates fluid where air should be, or consolidation in the lung field. The sound is picked up as air flows through the bronchi surrounding the alveoli filled with fluid.

Functional capacity

Functional capacity can be estimated directly by functional assessment and more indirectly by pulmonary function measurement (see Chapter 3). The functional assessment should include the patient's medical history of reported daily activity level (e.g., walks little, essentially bed to chair activities, walks 100 yards prior to shortness of breath). This information should be evaluated in relation to the actual functional measurement done during the initial patient evaluation. The type of evaluation of functional ability can vary greatly from the patient who is on mechanical ventilatory support to the non-intubated patient who is exercising regularly. The short-term ventilated patient usually does not need a functional assessment while ventilated. The focus of the functional evaluation should be on the patient who will require long-term ventilation. However, at times, it is difficult to foresee how long ventilatory support will be required, and patients may not receive the necessary early evaluation. The evaluation should include range of motion of the extremities and ability to move about without undue respiratory distress, including observation of increased respiratory rate if on intermittent ventilation, change in colour and undue increase in heart rate. The patient may also be directed towards an exercise programme to facilitate

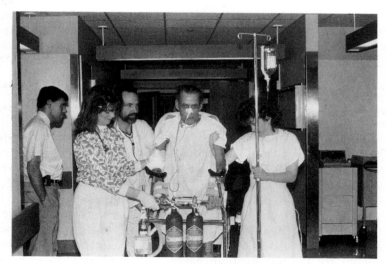

Figure 2.14 *This man, although requiring long-term ventilatory support, is now able to breathe independently with oxygen therapy while walking with assistance. Individuals still requiring ventilatory support may also be ambulated while being 'ambued' (bagged) or placed on a portable ventilatory support.*

weaning from a ventilator, and the evaluation should include the patient's response to sitting, standing, and, if the patient's condition allows, walking (Figure 2.14). The evaluation should not only include objective measures of response (respiratory rate/heart rate) but should include the patient's sense of comfort. This may include use of a scale of perceived effort and an adapted scale for dyspnoea.

The patient who has longstanding lung disease or debilitation requires a functional evaluation that would also include a few activities of daily living, such as ability to dress without limiting sense of dyspnoea. The six-minute walk test may be used to evaluate exercise capacity in preparation for a conditioning programme. The six-minute walk is done at the patient's own rate of ambulation, and the distance covered is recorded and used as a comparison after the conditioning programme. If the patient feels dyspnoeic, a rest is allowed, and the total distance covered in the six minutes is recorded.

SUMMARY

The clinician who reads a chart and establishes a treatment plan without a thorough assessment of the patient at the bedside may be delivering a treatment that is inappropriate to the patient, not indicated, or unnecessary. Careful patient assessment provides the information for an appropriate treatment plan and subsequent evaluation of treatment. These tools are critical to the clinician as they help ensure optimum patient care.

FURTHER READING

Bates B. (1991). *A Guide to Physical Examination and History Taking*. Philadelphia: J.B. Lippincott.

Kraman S.S. (1986). Lung sounds for the clinician. *Arch. Intern. Med.*, **146,** 1411.

Loudon R.G. (1987). The lung examination. *Clin. Chest. Med.*, **8,** 265.

Murray J.F., Nadel J.A. (1988). *Textbook of Respiratory Medicine*. Philadelphia: W.B. Saunders.

Stevens S.A., Becker K.L. (1988). How to perform picture-perfect respiratory assessment. *Nursing,* **18,** 57.

Chapter 3

Pulmonary Function Tests: Performance and Interpretation

JENNIFER ALISON

INTRODUCTION

Pulmonary function tests provide a guide to the state and function of the respiratory system. They are useful for distinguishing a healthy respiratory system from a diseased or damaged one; for assessing the degree of disease or disability; for monitoring the progress of disease and for measuring the response to treatment. Some pulmonary function tests are used by physiotherapists as part of the management of persons with respiratory disorders. There are many other tests, which are not currently administered by physiotherapists but may be in the future. A knowledge of the tests, how they are performed and an understanding of the information they provide assists the physiotherapist to make an informed contribution to the management of the patient.

SPIROMETRY

Spirometry is one of the most commonly performed tests of pulmonary function and is often carried out by a physiotherapist. It is the measurement of a single forced expiration from total lung capacity using a spirometer (Figure 3.1). It is a simple test which gives a great deal of information. The equipment is usually portable and the test is used regularly in hospital wards, outpatient departments and in community practice.

To perform the test the subject takes in as big a breath as possible and then blows out as hard and as fast and as long as possible into a spirometer. This results in a trace similar to that shown in Figure 3.2. From this trace three measurements can be made:

1 The amount of air that can be blown out in the first second of the forced expiration. This is known as the *forced expiratory volume in one second* (FEV_1). It is a measurement of the *flow rate* at which the air can be blown out from the lungs.
2 The *total* amount of air that can be blown out after a maximal inspiration.

This is known as the *vital capacity* (VC). If the measurement of VC occurs during a *forced* expiration it is called a *forced vital capacity* (FVC). The VC is a *volume* measurement.

3   The flow rate over the middle half of the expiratory curve. This is known as the *maximum mid-expiratory flow rate* (MMEFR, also known as $FEF_{25-75\%}$, that is, the mean forced expiratory flow between 25% and 75% of the vital capacity). The MMEFR is a *flow rate* measurement. Unfortunately it is not measured as routinely as FEV_1 and FVC although it is useful for early detection of changes in the small airways.

An important relationship exists between FEV_1 and FVC. An adult with normal lungs and normal respiratory muscles can blow out at least 79% of their vital capacity within the first second of expiration, that is, the FEV_1/FVC ratio expressed as a percentage is at least 79%. An FEV_1/FVC ratio of at least 79% indicates that there is not likely to be any significant obstruction to the flow of air out of the lungs. (In children this value should be nearer 100%.) The remaining 21% of air is usually blown out within the next two seconds so that a normal trace has a distinctive character and will be virtually flat after three seconds (Figure 3.2).

The FEV_1, FVC, FEV_1/FVC and MMEFR can be abnormal for a variety of reasons.

The FEV_1 is considered abnormal if it is 20% lower than the predicted normal value.

A reduction in FEV_1 can occur due to:

1   Narrowing of the airways. Even with maximum effort, the same volume of air cannot be pushed out as quickly through narrowed tubes. There are four main reasons why the airways may be narrowed (Figure 3.3):
     (a)   There may be spasm of the bronchial smooth muscle as occurs in asthma;

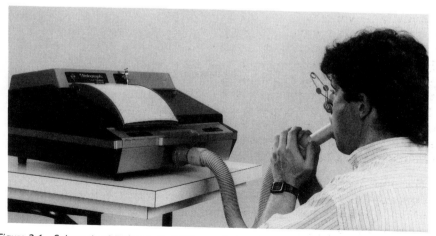

Figure 3.1   Spirometer (Vitalograph). (With permission FSE Scientific, Australia.)

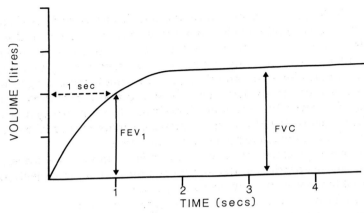

Figure 3.2   Normal spirometry trace showing the forced expiratory volume in one second (FEV$_1$) and the forced vital capacity (FVC).

(b)   The airway wall may be thickened by oedema or by hypertrophy of the bronchial smooth muscle, both of which cause the lumen to be narrowed;

(c)   The lumen of the airway may be partly blocked by excessive secretions;

(d)   Outside the airway, the lung parenchyma may be partly destroyed (as occurs in emphysema) and the airways become narrowed due to loss of radial traction.

Any disorder in which the flow of air is 'obstructed' by the above is grouped under the heading *obstructive lung disease*. Such disorders include asthma, cystic fibrosis, bronchiectasis, emphysema, chronic bronchitis and chronic obstructive lung disease (a combination of chronic bronchitis and emphysema). Persons with chronic obstructive disorders are said to have chronic airflow limitation (CAL).

2   Loss of expiratory muscle power. FEV$_1$ is an effort-dependent measurement. If the respiratory muscles are weak, air cannot be forced out as

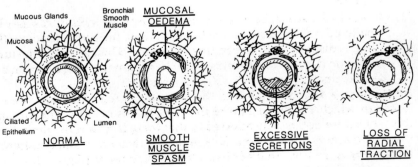

Figure 3.3   Schematic representation of a normal airway and causes of airway narrowing: spasm of the bronchial smooth muscle, mucosal oedema, excessive secretions and loss of radial traction.

quickly. This may occur in neuromuscular disorders such as Guillain–Barré syndrome, poliomyelitis, quadriplegia due to spinal cord injury. Muscle power may also be reduced to some extent when the lungs are hyperinflated (e.g., in emphysema, or in asthma during an attack) as hyperinflation alters the angle of pull and the resting length of the respiratory muscles so that they are working at a mechanical disadvantage. However, hyperinflation largely results from airway narrowing and the reduction in FEV_1 in such instances is more related to the narrow airways than to the altered muscle configuration.

3   Inadequate expiratory effort when there is no muscle weakness. This may occur due to lack of understanding on the part of the subject, pain or an unwillingness of the subject to cooperate.

4   Abnormal compressibility of the intrathoracic trachea.

The VC is considered abnormal if it is 20% less than predicted normal. *A reduction in VC can occur due to:*

1   Factors that reduce inspiration. VC is largely dependent on the volume of air that can be *inhaled* before a maximal expiration, therefore anything that diminishes this will reduce VC. Disorders in which this occurs include:

(a)   Chest wall deformities such as those that can occur as a consequence of scoliosis. The lungs are compressed due to the deformed rib cage so their volume is reduced. (In addition, the respiratory muscles are working at a mechanical disadvantage.)

(b)   Neuromuscular disorders, e.g., Guillain–Barré syndrome, quadriplegia due to spinal cord injury, poliomyelitis. In such cases both inspiratory and expiratory muscle power is diminished. If the person can only breathe in a small volume of air due to loss of muscle power then the amount blown out will also be reduced.

(c)   Pleural disease, e.g., pleural effusion where fluid collects in the pleural cavity. If there is a large amount of fluid it will compress the lung and thus reduce its volume, consequently VC will be reduced.

(d)   Interstitial disease. In such diseases the airways themselves may be unaltered but the lung parenchyma, that is, the actual tissue of the lung, is diseased, often resulting in fibrosis. This can make the lung 'stiff' and difficult to expand so that the volume of air the person can inhale, and consequently exhale, is reduced.

All the above disorders fall into the category of *restrictive lung diseases* (those in which the expansion of the lung is 'restricted'). The airways themselves are not usually affected in that there is no airflow limitation, that is, no airway obstruction. Such diseases result in a totally different spirometry trace from that of obstructive lung disease (Figure 3.4).

2   Factors that limit the amount and/or the flow of air expired. This occurs in such disorders as:

(a) Airway obstruction (e.g., in asthma) where narrowed airways cause early airway closure during expiration. Less air is expelled, consequently the VC is smaller. The air that is not expelled remains in the lungs at the end of maximal expiration resulting in an increased residual volume (see Lung Volumes).

(b) Loss of lung recoil or elasticity (e.g., in emphysema) where once again the airways close early in expiration, limiting the amount of air that can be expelled.

Examination of the FEV_1/FVC ratio provides additional information. As already stated, the FEV_1/FVC ratio is normally greater than or equal to 79%. When there is airway obstruction the FEV_1/FVC ratio is always less than 79%. In other words, a smaller proportion of the total amount of air can be blown out in the first second through obstructed airways. The FEV_1/FVC ratio gives a measure of the degree of airway obstruction and can be as low as 20%. An example of the spirometry trace of a person with airway obstruction (Figure 3.4) shows that it takes much longer than three seconds to blow all the air out and that the proportion blown out in the first second is small in relation to the total amount.

In restrictive lung disease, even though the FEV_1 and FVC may be reduced from normal, the FEV_1/FVC ratio is preserved or increased. This is because there is no narrowing of the airways so there is no obstruction to airflow. The small amount of air that is inhaled can be expelled quickly (Figure 3.4), sometimes aided by an increase in elastic recoil observed in some restrictive lung diseases.

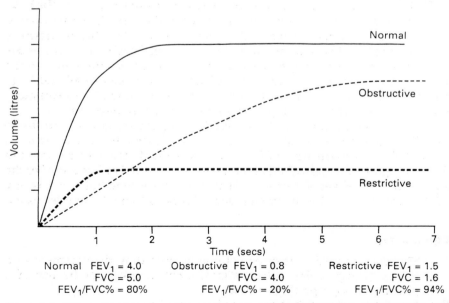

Normal FEV$_1$ = 4.0	Obstructive FEV$_1$ = 0.8	Restrictive FEV$_1$ = 1.5
FVC = 5.0	FVC = 4.0	FVC = 1.6
FEV$_1$/FVC% = 80%	FEV$_1$/FVC% = 20%	FEV$_1$/FVC% = 94%

Figure 3.4 Spirometry traces from the normal lung and from obstructive and restrictive lung disease.

NORMAL   AIRWAY

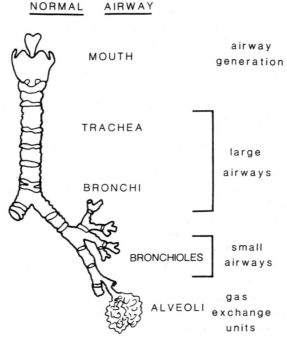

Figure 3.5   Schematic representation of airway generations indicating the distinction between the large and small airways.

The FEF$_{25-75\%}$ is reduced in airways disease for the same reasons as the FEV$_1$ is reduced. However, in some instances when the FEV$_1$ is within normal limits the FEF$_{25-75\%}$ may be reduced. This can be an early indicator of airway disease since the FEF$_{25-75\%}$ measures flow in the smaller airways where early changes are more detectable, whereas the FEV$_1$ is a measure of flow in the larger airways. Figure 3.5 shows the distinction between small and large airways. The FEF$_{25-75\%}$ correlates well with the maximum mid-expiratory flow ($\dot{V}_{50}$) measurement of the flow-volume curve (see page 36).

FEV$_1$ and FVC are measured to assess the progress of a disease and also to establish the effect of treatment. In a person hospitalized with asthma, twice-daily measurements of FEV$_1$ and FVC should ideally be recorded to follow progress. FEV$_1$ and FVC should also be measured before and after the administration of aerosol bronchodilator to assess whether there is any acute reversibility of the obstruction due to bronchial smooth muscle spasm.

Equipment

(a)   Spirometer which measures volume by recording displacement of a wedge (Figure 3.6a), a bell (Figure 3.6b), a piston or by use of a pneumotachograph (Figure 3.6c).
(b)   Nose clip and mouthpiece.
(c)   Spirometer paper.

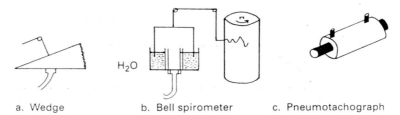

H₂O

a. Wedge   b. Bell spirometer   c. Pneumotachograph

Figure 3.6 Methods of measuring volumes of gas: (a) wedge in which air enters a wedge bellows and causes displacement of a recording needle; (b) bell spirometer in which air enters the bell causing it to rise in the water which displaces a recording pen on a chymograph; (c) pneumotachograph from which the flow of gas is recorded and integrated to give volume.

Procedure

(a) Explain the reason for the test and the test procedure.

(b) Ask the subject to loosen tight clothing (especially tight-fitting collar, necktie, brassiere or belt).

(c) Subject may be seated or standing.

(d) The mouthpiece should be positioned so that the chin is slightly elevated and the neck extended.

(e) Apply nose clip.

(f) Instruct the subject to take a *maximal* breath in from a normal breathing pattern, put the mouthpiece in the mouth with the lips tightly around it and then to blow out as *hard* and as *fast* and *completely* as possible into the spirometer. The head position, with the chin slightly elevated, should be maintained throughout the test.

(g) Encourage the subject throughout the manoeuvre to perform maximally.

(h) The operator should ensure that the paper is moving at the appropriate speed during the manoeuvre.

(i) The performance of the manoeuvre should be evaluated and instructions given again if necessary. Possible problems may be:
   (i) loss of air before the mouthpiece is properly in place;
   (ii) leaking around the mouthpiece during the test;
   (iii) coughing throughout the manoeuvre;
   (iv) inability to sustain an expiration for five seconds;
   (v) less than maximum effort both on inspiration and expiration on the part of the subject.

(j) Ideally three reproducible acceptable tracings should be obtained.

Individuals with severe obstructive lung disease take a long time to expel all the air, and expiration may continue for 20 seconds or more, unlike the 3–5 seconds in a normal person. Prolonged FVC efforts may cause syncopal episodes. It seems reasonable to stop the FVC manoeuvre after 10 seconds unless terminated earlier because of dyspnoea or lightheadedness.

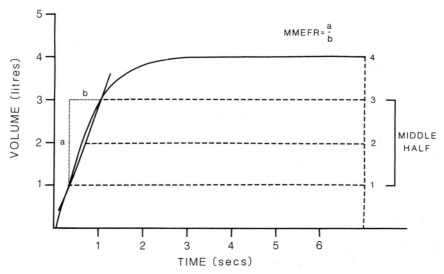

Figure 3.7   Calculation of maximum mid-expiratory flow rate (MMEFR). Also known as $FEF_{25-75\%}$.

Calculations

The measurements obtained from the spirometry trace are the FEV_1 and the FVC (see Figure 3.2). It is acceptable to record the largest FEV_1 and the largest FVC from the three best traces even if the values do not come from the same curve. The FEV_1/FVC percentage is then calculated. The $FEF_{25-75\%}$ is calculated as in Figure 3.7. To be able to calculate the $FEF_{25-75\%}$ it is necessary to have a trace for the total time of the manoeuvre. If a person cannot exhale all the air within the time scale of the spirometer chart an extrapolation will need to be made. Alternatively, the measurement may be done on a bell spirometer where there is no limit to the time scale. The $FEF_{25-75\%}$ is calculated using the best of the three spirometry traces. The best single trace is considered to be that with largest sum of FEV_1 and FVC.

All measurements are made in ambient temperature and pressure, saturated (ATPS) and converted to body temperature and pressure, saturated (BTPS) for recording in the patient's notes. Conversions of ATPS and BTPS are given in Jones et al.[1]

Normal Values

Normal values for VC have been provided by studies of large numbers of subjects without symptoms of lung disease and are related to the subject's age, height and sex. For adults these values are given by Grimby and Soderholm,[2] and for children by Polgar and Promadhat.[3] A guideline for a predictive equation for normal values is given in Table 3.1. For FEV_1 normal values are calculated as 79% of the predicted VC.

TABLE 3.1

Prediction equations for lung volumes, spirometry, maximum inspiratory mouth pressures (Pimax), maximum expiratory mouth pressures (Pemax), partial pressure of arterial oxygen (Pao₂), partial pressure of arterial carbon dioxide (Paco₂) and hydrogen ion concentration (pH) in normal healthy adults (SEE = standard error of the estimate)

Index	Sex	Regression Coefficients Height(cm)	Age(yr)	Constant term	SEE	Source
Total lung capacity	F	0.0590		−4.537	0.536	10
(litres BTPS)	M	0.0795	+0.0032	−7.333	0.792	
Functional residual	F	0.0360	+0.0031	−3.182	0.523	10
capacity (litres BTPS)	M	0.0472	+0.0090	−5.290	0.718	
Residual volume	F	0.0197	+0.0201	−2.421	0.381	10
(litres BTPS)	M	0.0216	+0.0207	−2.840	0.374	
Forced vital capacity	F	0.0491	−0.0216	−3.590	0.393	16
(litres BTPS)	M	0.0600	−0.0214	−4.650	0.644	
Forced expiratory volume	F	0.0342	−0.0255	−1.578	0.326	16
1 sec (litres BTPS)	M	0.0414	−0.0244	−2.190	0.486	
P_{Imax}	F	0.71		−43		13
(cmH₂O)	M		−1.03	142		
P_{Emax}	F	0.55		3.5		13
(cmH₂O)	M		−0.91	180		
Pao₂ (mmHg)			−0.27	104.2		17
Paco₂ (mmHg)				36–44		18
pH				7.35–7.45		

Reproducibility

The variability of the test in normal subjects is approximately 10%. Persons with obstructive lung disease show greater variability than normal subjects.[4] There appears to be no diurnal variation in maximal flow.[5]

PEAK EXPIRATORY FLOW RATE

Peak expiratory flow rate (PEFR) is another simple test of lung function. It is the greatest, or peak, flow that can be generated by a subject when blowing air out of the lungs as explosively as possible following a maximum in-spiration. It is a very effort-dependent measurement. The PEFR is deter-mined by lung volume, the calibre of the airways and the elastic recoil of the lung. Since the PEFR is recorded at the beginning of expiration it has the advantage of not requiring a total forced expiration which can cause cough-ing. The measurement of PEFR can detect changes in airway calibre as may occur in asthma, chronic bronchitis, emphysema.

PEFR does not give as much information as spirometry. However, peak expiratory flow meters (Figure 3.8) are compact, portable, easy to use and inexpensive compared with spirometers, making the measurement of PEFR a commonly used test. The manoeuvre itself is so quick that the measurement of PEFR is more applicable than spirometry in some situations, for example, when measuring changes in airway calibre during exercise in asthmatic subjects.

In some restrictive lung diseases that affect the interstitial tissue, the PEFR may be within normal limits, or even high, although the lung volumes are reduced. The maintenance of PEFR can occur because the airways are not narrowed. In fact, due to increased radial traction, the airways' calibre may be large when related to lung volume (Figure 3.9), thus allowing high flows still to be generated. Flow rate may also be enhanced by an increase in elastic recoil observed in some restrictive lung diseases.

Equipment

(a) Peak flow meter. There are a number of peak flow meters available. The original peak flow meter was developed by Wright (see Figure 3.8). In this meter a vane is deflected by the flow of forcibly expired air. The angle of deflection is a function of the rate of gas flow. Other simple plastic devices such as the Wright Mini Peak Flow Meter and Allersearch Peak Flow Meter (see Figure 3.8) show good correlation with flow rates from the original Wright Peak Flow Meter.

(b) Mouthpiece.

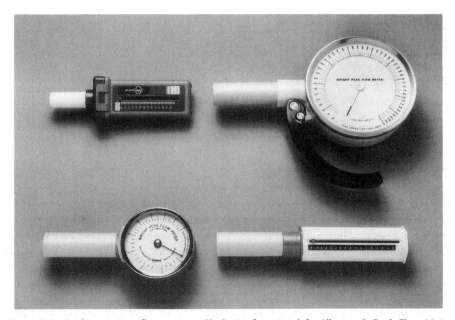

Figure 3.8   Peak expiratory flow meters. Clockwise from top left: Allersearch Peak Flow Meter (available in standard and low range), Wright Peak Flow Meter (adult), Wright Mini Peak Flow Meter, Wright Peak Flow Meter (children). (With permission Clarke International, Australia.)

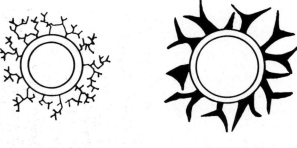

NORMAL   FIBROSIS

Figure 3.9   Diagrammatic representation of airway calibre in pulmonary fibrosis. Radial traction may be excessive, with the result that airway calibre is large when related to lung volume. (Modified from West J.B. Pulmonary Pathophysiology—the Essentials. *Baltimore: Williams & Wilkins. With permission from Williams & Wilkins © 1977.)*

Procedure

(a)   The subject is asked to take in the deepest breath possible, then to put the mouthpiece in the mouth and to give a short, sharp, fast, explosive blow into the meter.
(b)   The meter is reset to zero.
(c)   The test is repeated twice and the best of the three attempts is recorded.

Calculations

The value achieved is read directly from the meter in litres per minute.

Normal Values

The peak expiratory flow rate is related to a person's age, sex and height. Normal values in adults[6,7] and children[8] have been established by measuring the PEFR in normal subjects.

AIRFLOW METER READINGS

The Airflow Meter (Figure 3.10) is another device for assessing lung function and was developed as a low cost alternative to measuring PEFR or FEV_1. The airflow meter reading is influenced by the flow rate of exhaled air as well as by its volume and correlates well with FEV_1.[9] Since it is a low cost instrument and is light and portable, the airflow meter is generally used for individuals monitoring their daily lung function at home. By comparing the initial airflow meter reading with an FEV_1 reading taken at the same time, the relationship between FEV_1 and the airflow meter reading can be established for that person.

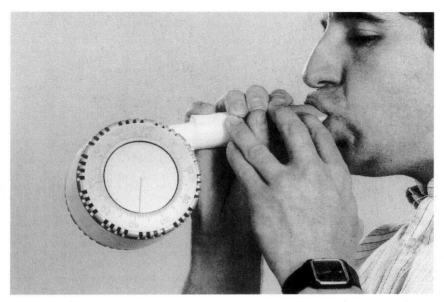

Figure 3.10   Airflow Meter.

Equipment

(a)   Airflow Meter.
(b)   Mouthpiece.

Procedure

(a)   The subject is asked to take a very big breath in and to blow out as hard and fast and as long as possible into the meter.
(b)   The dial will continue to turn even when the subject stops blowing. (The meter should be held in the horizontal plane.)
(c)   The meter is read when the dial stops turning.
(d)   The best of three measurements is recorded.

Calculation

The reading is taken directly from the meter and is recorded in airflow meter (AFM) units. One revolution is 100 AFM units.

FLOW-VOLUME LOOP

The maximal flow-volume loop of the lung shows graphically changes in expiratory and inspiratory flow rates with changes in lung volume (from total lung capacity to residual volume and vice-versa). In a person with

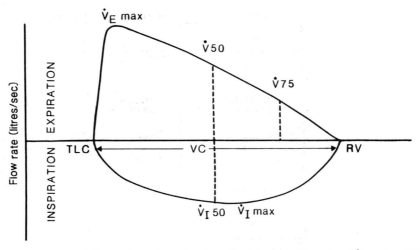

Figure 3.11   Normal flow–volume loop showing maximum expiratory flow ($\dot{V}_E$max) which is equivalent to the peak expiratory flow rate (PEFR), maximum expiratory flow rate at 50% VC (V_{50}), maximum expiratory flow rate at 75% VC ($\dot{V}_{75}$), maximum inspiratory flow ($\dot{V}_I$max), maximum inspiratory flow rate at 50% VC ($\dot{V}_I$max$_{50}$). TLC = total lung capacity; RV = residual volume; VC = vital capacity.

normal lungs and normal respiratory muscles the loop has a characteristic shape and looks like a triangle sitting on a semi-circle (Figure 3.11). The expiratory part of the flow-volume loop is called the *flow-volume curve*.

The shape of the flow-volume loop provides a good visual guide to changes in the respiratory system and allows easier recognition of some abnormalities especially those confined to the large central airways and the small airways. Abnormal narrowing of the large central airways such as the larynx or trachea produces a characteristic pattern on the expiratory portion of the flow-volume loop. There is a restriction of peak flow and a plateau of flow at high lung volumes (Figure 3.12b). Such narrowing may occur in strictures of the trachea (e.g., following intubation), malignant neoplasms, bilateral vocal cord paralysis. Obstruction of small peripheral airways may cause a reduction in flow at low lung volumes which is readily detected from the concave shape of the flow-volume curve. Such changes are usually overlooked in standard analysis of spirometry. The reduction in flow may occur immediately expiration begins resulting in an abrupt fall after the peak flow is reached. This is known as pressure-dependent collapse of the airways and occurs in emphysema (Figure 3.12c). Alternatively, the airways may collapse progressively with expiration resulting in a more gradual scooping out of the expiratory curve. This is known as volume-dependent collapse and is more common in asthma (Figure 3.12d).

A particular characteristic of the descending portion of the flow-volume curve is that this part of the curve *in any one individual* takes virtually the same path no matter how great an expiratory effort is made. The implication is that despite a wide range of expiratory effort the flow rate cannot be

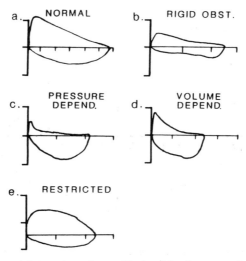

Figure 3.12   Examples of flow–volume loops. (Horizontal axis represents volume; vertical axis represents flow.)

altered at mid or low lung volumes, that is, flow is independent of maximal effort. This is called the *effort-independent* part of the curve (Figure 3.13). The reason for this occurring is that during forced expiration a pressure gradient down the airway is established. At some point the pressure inside the lumen of the airway equals the pleural pressure (i.e., the pressure surrounding the wall of the airway). This is called the equal pressure point (EPP) (Figure 3.14). Downstream from this point (i.e., towards the mouth) compression of the airway develops. Under these conditions the pressure gradient between the alveolus and the equal pressure point is equal to the elastic recoil pressure (Pel). Thus airflow occurs due to the elastic recoil pressure and is limited by the resistance offered by the airways from the alveolus to the compression point. Therefore, after the equal pressure point is reached,

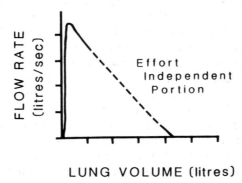

Figure 3.13   Flow–volume curve. The broken line represents the effort-independent portion of the curve. (Modified from West J.B. Respiratory Physiology—the Essentials*. Baltimore: Williams & Wilkins. With permission from Williams & Wilkins © 1974.)*

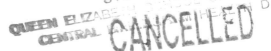

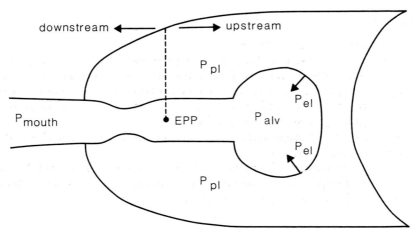

Figure 3.14 *A diagrammatic representation of the equal pressure point (EPP) concept. At the EPP the pressure inside the airway equals the pleural pressure (P_{pl}) i.e., the pressure outside the airway. Downstream from this point airway compression occurs and the driving force for airflow becomes the elastic recoil pressure (P_{el}).*

maximum expiratory flow is determined by the physical properties of the lung alone, and increases in expiratory effort will not increase airflow, that is, flow is independent of the subject's effort. It is the effort-independent part of the curve that represents the *characteristic* of the lung tissue. For example, in emphysema the effort-independent part of the curve is very flat since only low flows can be maintained after the equal pressure point is reached because of loss of elastic recoil (see Figure 3.12c). However, in some restrictive lung diseases where the lungs are stiff, higher flows are maintained at lower lung volumes and the flow-volume curve is maintained or even convex because of the increased elastic recoil and more rigid airways (see Figure 3.12e).

During inspiration the above considerations do not apply as the walls of the airways are pulled apart rather than compressed. Therefore, inspiratory flow is relatively dependent upon the power of the inspiratory muscles (the diaphragm and intercostals). Inspiratory flow will be reduced in neuromuscular disorders or if there is poor effort from the subject. Extrathoracic airway obstruction will also result in a reduced inspiratory flow (see Figure 3.12b).

Equipment

(a) Either a flow-meter (pneumotachograph), or volume-meter, or both. If a flow-meter is used then the flow signal is integrated to obtain respired volume. If a volume-meter is used by itself, the volume signal is differentiated to obtain flow.

(b) X–Y recorder, which plots flow and volume signals.

(c) Mouthpiece.

Procedure

(a)–(e) the same as for spirometry.

(f)   The subject is instructed to take in the deepest breath possible, to put the mouthpiece in the mouth with the lips tightly around, on a given signal to blow out as hard and fast as possible until no more air can be squeezed out, and, finally, to breathe back in again as fast as possible until the lungs are maximally inflated.

(g)   The operator should encourage the subject throughout the test to ensure maximal effort.

(h)   The performance of the manoeuvre should be evaluated and the subject's technique should be corrected if necessary. Possible problems may be the same as (i) in spirometry.

Calculations

A number of respiratory measurements can be read from the trace (see Figure 3.11). Those most commonly derived are:

(a)   Maximum expiratory flow—$\dot{V}_E max$ which is the PEFR.

(b)   Maximum mid-expiratory flow, i.e. the flow at 50% of the VC—$\dot{V}_E max_{50}$ which is abbreviated to $\dot{V}_{50}$ (also known as $FEF_{50\%}$). This equates well to $FEF_{25-75\%}$.

(c)   Late expiratory flow—$\dot{V}_E max_{75}$ or $\dot{V}_{75}$.

(d)   Peak inspiratory flow—$\dot{V}_I max$.

(e)   Maximum mid-inspiratory flow—$\dot{V}_I max_{50}$.

Normal Values

Normal values for the maximal expiratory flow-volume curve are given by Knudson and colleagues.[5]

LUNG VOLUMES

The volume of gas in the lungs can be measured at fixed points during the breathing cycle. These are known as static lung volumes. The measurement of lung volumes is valuable in the detection and diagnosis of diseases affecting the lungs and also in monitoring the natural history or the response to treatment of such diseases. The principal static lung volumes are total lung capacity (TLC), functional residual capacity (FRC) and residual volume (RV) (Figure 3.15).

The *total lung capacity* (TLC) is the total amount of gas that the lungs can hold at the end of a maximal inspiration. When all the air is blown out of the lungs by active and prolonged expiration, some air still remains no matter how much effort is made to expel it. The amount that remains is called the

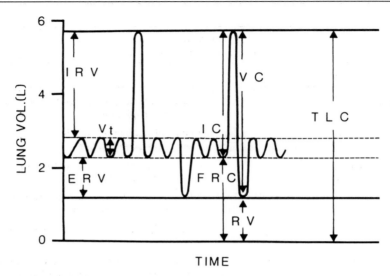

Figure 3.15   Lung volumes. TLC = total lung capacity; RV = residual volume; FRC = functional residual capacity; VC = vital capacity; IC = inspiratory capacity; IRV = inspiratory reserve volume; ERV = expiratory reserve volume; V_t = tidal volume.

residual volume (RV). Similarly, during normal tidal breathing a volume of gas remains in the lungs at the end of quiet expiration. This is known as the *function residual capacity* (FRC) because it is the *functioning* residual volume. It is this volume of air which is used in the continued transfer of oxygen and carbon dioxide into and out of the blood between periods of inspiration. RV and FRC cannot be measured using direct breathing manoeuvres. These volumes can be measured indirectly either by gas dilution or body plethysmography.

Measurements of lung volumes that can be made directly are the *inspiratory capacity* (IC) which is the volume of air that can be inhaled following a quiet expiration, and the *vital capacity* (VC). Once the IC, FRC and VC are known the other lung volumes, TLC and RV, can be derived. Figure 3.15 shows the lung volumes as they appear on a spirogram. Table 3.2 gives a description of the lung volumes.

There are three methods of measuring lung volumes—helium dilution, body plethysmography and radiographic estimation.

Helium Dilution Technique for Measuring Lung Volumes

This method is used to measure RV or FRC by dilution of a marker gas in the unknown lung volume of the thorax. It relies on the principle that in a closed system the initial volume of gas (V_1) multiplied by the initial concentration of the marker gas (C_1) equals the final volume of gas (V_2) multiplied by the final concentration of the marker gas (C_2), i.e., $V_1 \times C_1 = V_2 \times C_2$. Helium is now

TABLE 3.2
Description of lung volumes and capacities

Lung volume or capacity	Description
Total lung capacity	Total amount of gas contained in the lung at maximal inspiration
Functional residual capacity	Volume of gas that remains in the lungs at the end of resting expiration
Residual volume	Volume of gas that remains in the lungs at the end of maximal expiration
Vital capacity	Total volume of gas that can be expired following a maximal inspiration
Inspiratory capacity	Volume of gas inspired from the end of resting expiration
Inspiratory reserve volume	Maximum volume of gas that can be inspired from the end of resting inspiration
Expiratory reserve volume	Maximum volume of gas that can be expired from the end of resting expiration
Tidal volume	Volume of gas inspired or expired during each breathing cycle

most commonly used as a marker gas because it is insoluble in blood and hence mixes only with the gas in the lungs.

Equipment

(a) Rolling seal spirometer equipped with a blower to mix helium and air, and a soda lime canister to absorb carbon dioxide (CO_2). The spirometer should be capable of recording an inspiratory capacity of at least five litres.
(b) A thermal conductivity helium meter which is connected in the circuit so that all sampled gas returns to the system.
(c) Tank of 100% O_2 to supplement O_2 loss.

Procedure

(a) Explanation to the subject of the overall test procedure.
(b) The subject is seated comfortably with a flanged mouthpiece in the mouth and a nose clip in place.
(c) If *FRC is to be measured* the subject is asked to breathe room air normally. At the end of a quiet, tidal expiration the operator turns the mouthpiece valve so that the subject now breathes only from the spirometer. The spirometer contains a known concentration of helium (C_1) mixed with air. The volume of gas in the spirometer is also a known volume (V_1).

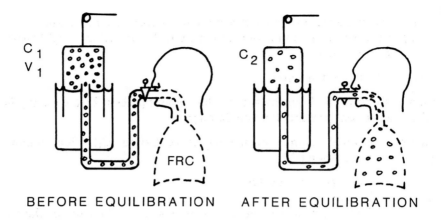

$$V_1 \times C_1 = (V_1 + FRC) \times C_2$$

Figure 3.16 Diagrammatic representation of the measurement of functional residual capacity by the helium dilution method. (Modified from West J.B. Respiratory Physiology—the Essentials. Baltimore: Williams & Wilkins. With permission from Williams & Wilkins © 1974.)

The helium is now able to mix with the volume of gas in the lungs, that is, with the FRC. The FRC will dilute the concentration of helium to a new concentration (C_2). The subject continues to breathe the helium and air mixture until the helium is thoroughly mixed with this new accessible gas volume. At this point the reading on the helium meter should be steady. The new, more dilute concentration of helium (C_2) is then recorded (Figure 3.16).

(d) The subject, while connected to the spirometer, is also asked to take in the biggest breath possible and then to blow out as much as possible. This gives a measure of IC and VC.

(e) While the subject is breathing from the spirometer, CO_2 is absorbed by the soda lime and the oxygen being used is replaced via a tube from the oxygen cylinder into the bell.

(f) If RV is to be measured, the procedure is the same as for the measurement of FRC, however, the operator connects the subject to the bell after the subject has breathed out as far as possible, that is, when the volume of gas in the lungs is the RV. The FRC method is used much more commonly than RV because it is more reproducible.

Calculations

(a) The IC and VC can be measured directly from the spirometer trace.
(b) To calculate the FRC:

The following values are known:

(i) the initial volume of helium and air mixture in the spirometer (V_1);

(ii)   the initial concentration of helium in the spirometer (C_1); and
(iii) the final concentration of helium when it has mixed thoroughly with the FRC (C_2).

The FRC is the unknown value:

Since no helium is lost from the system the amount present before mixing is equal to the amount present after equilibration.

Therefore, the initial volume (V_1) × initial concentration (C_1) = final volume (V_2) × final concentration (C_2)

V_1, C_1 and C_2 are all known values.
N.B. $V_2 = V_1 + FRC$
since $V_1 + FRC$ is the total volume that dilutes the helium to get the C_2 reading.

Therefore:

$$V_1 \times C_1 = (V_1 + FRC) \times C_2$$
$$V_1.C_1 = V_1.C_2 + FRC.C_2$$
$$V_1.C_1 - V_1.C_2 = FRC.C_2$$
$$V_1 \frac{(C_1 - C_2)}{C_2} = FRC$$

Now the known values are:

IC, VC and FRC.

From these, the remaining volumes can be calculated. Look at Figure 3.15 and see that:

IC + FRC = TLC
TLC − VC = RV

Now all the lung volumes are known.

The lung volumes are initially calculated in ATPS and should be converted to BTPS to give a correct reading. Normal values are reported in litres BTPS.

Normal Values

Normal values for lung volumes measured by helium dilution technique are given by Crapo and colleagues[10] and Grimby and Soderholm.[2] Regression relationships for predicting lung volumes appear in Table 3.1.

Total Body Plethysmography for Measuring Lung Volumes

This is another method of measuring lung volumes in which the subject is seated inside a body plethysmograph which is a large, airtight box often

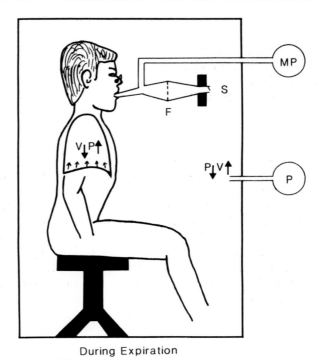

During Expiration

Figure 3.17 Measurement of functional residual capacity using a constant volume body plethys-mograph. V = volume; P = pressure; F = flow-meter or pneumotachygraph; S = shutter; MP = mouth pressure gauge.

called a 'body box' (Figure 3.17). In most laboratories the constant-volume variable-pressure type plethysmograph, known as a pressure box, is used. The subject is asked to attempt to inspire and expire (i.e. pant) against a closed shutter when the volume of gas in the lungs is close to FRC. During panting the gas volume in the lungs is alternately compressed and expanded by the action of the respiratory muscles while changes in mouth pressures and box pressures are recorded. During the expiratory phase of panting, for example, the compression of gas in the lungs allows the air in the plethysmograph to expand slightly and its pressure falls since pressure × volume is constant in a closed system. The pressure sensor attached to the plethysmograph measures the changes in box pressure which reflects changes in thoracic volume. The pressure sensor attached to the mouthpiece senses the mouth pressure which is equal to the alveolar pressure developed in doing this manoeuvre. Since changes in thoracic volume and alveolar pressure can be measured and body fluids are incompressible, the volume of gas in the thoraco-abdominal cavity (thoracic gas volume) can be calculated by applying Boyle's Law, that is, pressure × volume is constant (PV = K) at constant temperature.

Equipment

(a) Semi-rigid, airtight 'body box'.
(b) Mouthpiece, shutter and noseclip.
(c) Pressure transducers.
(d) Oscilloscope or XY recorder.

Procedure

(a) Explain to the subject the overall test procedure.
(b) Seat the subject inside the box and demonstrate the shutter mechanism and panting technique.
(c) Encourage the subject to relax the chest during tidal breathing so that the end-tidal point will represent the subject's usual FRC.
(d) Adjust nose clip and mouthpiece, close the door and vent the box.
(e) Wait until the subject is settled and breathing quietly then at end-expiration ask the subject to pant lightly against a closed shutter.
(f) Record changes in pressure at the mouth and in the box during the panting manoeuvre.

Calculations

Boyle's Law states that $P \times V = $ constant at constant temperature. This can also be written as $P_1 \times V_1 = P_2 \times V_2$. When the subject makes an expiratory effort against the closed shutter the volume in the lungs is reduced by increasing airway pressure. This is recorded as an increase in mouth pressure. There is now more space in the box and the box pressure falls. By knowing the change in pressure of the box and its volume, the change in volume of the lung (ΔV) can be calculated. Boyle's Law is then applied to the air in the lungs by using the equation $P_1 \times V_1 = P_2 \times (V_1 - \Delta V)$ where V_1 is the FRC and P_1 and P_2 are the mouth pressures. From this the thoracic gas volume, which is an approximate of FRC, can be calculated.

This plethysmographic measurement also includes abdominal gas volume which has been estimated to average 130 ml. Accordingly, this volume may be subtracted from the plethysmographic result.

Normal Values

Normal values for lung volumes measured by plethysmography are derived from gas dilution techniques.[2,10]

Comparison of Helium Dilution and Body Plethysmography Techniques as Measurements of Lung Volumes

The helium dilution technique measures the *accessible* gas volume, that is, the volume of gas that can be reached by the helium during the time of the test. This gives a fairly accurate measurement of lung volumes and is usually similar to those measured by body plethysmography. In some instances, however, where areas of lung are not well ventilated (e.g., in severe airway obstruction), or where areas are not ventilated at all (e.g., lung cysts) the lung volume measured by helium dilution is less than that measured by body plethysmography. This is because body plethysmography measures the total volume of gas in the lungs including any trapped behind closed airways. The difference in measurements by the two methods can indicate the degree of air trapping or the size of the lung cyst.

Radiographic Estimates of Lung Volumes

A third method of measuring lung volumes is by use of chest X-rays. Postero-anterior and lateral films are taken when the subject is at maximum inspiration (i.e., TLC). The lung volume is estimated by direct measurement of the physical images.

This method has the advantage that it requires very little cooperation from the subject and can make use of radiographs taken for other purposes. However, it has not been established whether this technique is sufficiently accurate as a clinically useful measurement of TLC in individual patients. Its main role may be in retrospective or serial studies of trends in lung volumes where absolute accuracy is not essential.[11]

Interpreting Results of Lung Volume Measurements

The comparison of measured lung volumes with predicted normal values gives useful information for clinical diagnosis as well as for understanding functional problems.

If the TLC and/or FRC are greater than 120% of predicted normal the subject is said to have hyperinflated lungs. This is indicative of obstructive lung disease such as emphysema, or asthma during an exacerbation. In such instances, more air than normal remains in the lungs at the end of expiration due to early airway closure because of narrowed airways or loss of radial traction. Figure 3.18 shows a lung volume trace in a subject with obstructive lung disease. If the RV alone is greater than 120% of predicted normal and TLC and FRC are within normal limits this is an indication of gas trapping.

Alternatively, if the FRC, RV and TLC are less than 80% of the predicted normal values the subject is said to have small lung volumes which is indicative of restrictive lung disease, for example, pulmonary fibrosis (Figure 3.18).

As well as distinguishing obstructive and restrictive lung disease, lung volume measurements are useful in following the natural history of a disease and are also helpful in monitoring the effect of treatment. For example, treatment of obstructive lung disease may be aimed at decreasing hyperinflation, that is, getting RV and FRC back towards normal. Serial measurements of lung volumes will indicate if treatment is being effective. Reducing hyperinflation returns the chest to a more advantageous configuration for respiratory muscle work and hence reduces the work of breathing. Changes in hyperinflation cannot easily be gauged by other methods such as spirometry.

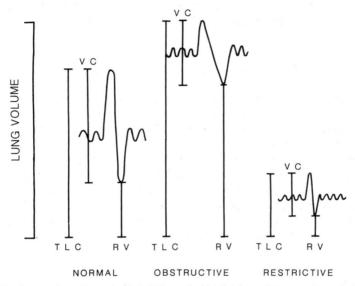

Figure 3.18   *Lung volume traces in obstructive and restrictive lung disease compared with normal.*

MAXIMAL INSPIRATORY AND EXPIRATORY MOUTH PRESSURES

The respiratory muscles and the chest wall provide the pressure pump to move gas in and out of the lungs. Consequently they are vitally important to lung function. Paralysis of the respiratory muscles, as can occur in quadriplegia or Guillain–Barré syndrome, may result in death unless artificial means are used to ventilate the lung.

Unlike limb skeletal muscles, the strength of the respiratory muscles cannot be measured directly. A simple, indirect means of measuring respiratory muscle strength is the measurement of the pressure generated at the mouth during maximum inspiratory and expiratory efforts against a closed valve.

The evaluation of inspiratory muscle strength by measuring *maximal inspiratory pressure* ($P_I$max) is useful in the diagnosis and management of persons with neuromuscular disease or with injuries involving the inspiratory muscles, that is, diaphragm, intercostals and accessory muscles. In both cases the available muscle power is decreased. $P_I$max is also useful for evaluating individuals whose strength of inspiration is reduced secondary to hyperinflation (e.g., emphysema). The hyperinflation alters the length/tension relationship of the respiratory muscles. Severe chest wall deformities, which may occur in scoliosis, also alter the length/tension relationship of the respiratory muscles and can cause a reduction in muscle strength at particular muscle lengths.

Measurement of $P_I$max is often used to indicate when patients can be successfully weaned from ventilators. Prolonged artificial ventilation, when inspiratory muscles were initially normal, may result in the muscles becoming weak from disuse. In such instances the muscles will need to be 'retrained' before the patient can be weaned from the ventilator. Alternatively, during recovery from a neuromuscular disease, measurement of inspiratory muscle strength may indicate when a patient can be successfully weaned from the ventilator.

$P_I$max is related to lung volume. It is maximal at residual volume (RV) and close to zero at total lung capacity (TLC). $P_I$max may be affected by changes in posture, being maximum in a forward sitting position and reduced in supine.

Expiration is normally a passive event. Failure of the expiratory muscles rarely causes respiratory failure as long as the inspiratory muscles are adequate. However, expiratory muscle strength is an important factor for an effective cough, therefore measurement of *maximal expiratory pressure* ($P_E$max) is often valuable in the evaluation of persons with impaired cough and retained secretions. $P_E$max is also used for the assessment of individuals with neuromuscular disorders. Large reductions in expiratory muscle strength may result in a reduced expiratory reserve volume and a reduction in expiratory flow rates which may be incorrectly interpreted as signs of obstructive airway disease. $P_E$max is related to lung volume. It is maximal at TLC and close to zero at RV.

The values recorded for $P_I$max and $P_E$max are directly affected by effort. It is therefore essential that the subjects be carefully instructed and co-operate fully. The pressure gauge for measuring $P_I$max and $P_E$max is portable so that it is possible to measure respiratory muscle strength at the bedside.

Equipment

(a)   Hand-held manometer capable of reading $\pm$ 200 cmH$_2$O (Figure 3.19).
(b)   One-way valve with a 2 mm leak hole. The leak hole is to prevent cheek muscles from providing significant pressures and thus distorting the pressures created by the respiratory muscles.
(c)   Flanged rubber mouthpiece.
(d)   Noseclip.

Procedure

1   $P_I$max
   (a)   Explain the procedure to the subject emphasizing the importance of maximum effort.
   (b)   Seat the subject upright with noseclip and mouthpiece in place.
   (c)   Instruct the subject to breathe all the way out (to RV) and then to make a maximal inspiratory effort against the closed valve for at least three seconds.
   (d)   Record the maximum negative inspiratory pressure sustained *after* the initial overshoot secondary to the inertia of the gauge needle or chest wall.
   (e)   Repeat the test until reproducible values are achieved to within $-5.0\,cmH_2O$, recording all values.
   (f)   Compare the best values with predicted normal.
2   $P_E$max
   (a)   Same as for $P_I$max except that the subject is instructed to breathe all the way in (to TLC) and then to make a maximal expiratory effort against the closed valve.
   (b)   The maximum expiratory pressure observed over 2–3 seconds is recorded (ignoring the initial needle overshoot).

The measurement of $P_E$max can be very uncomfortable due to the high pressures generated. In most instances it is only necessary to ascertain that the subject can generate a pressure of $100\,cmH_2O$ for men and $80\,cmH_2O$ for women as these values represent the lower limit of normal.

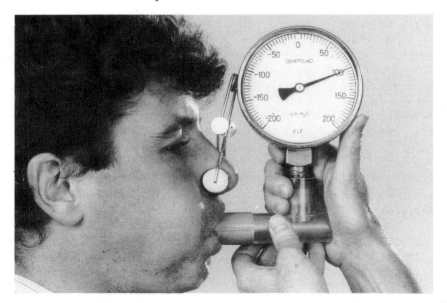

Figure 3.19   Hand-held pressure manometer for measuring inspiratory and expiratory mouth pressures. (With permission Record Instruments, Australia.)

Calculations

For $P_I$max report the most negative value of those recorded. For $P_E$max report the most positive value of those recorded.

Normal Values

Normal values are given in Wilson and colleagues,[12] and Black and Hyatt.[13] Predictive equations for $P_I$max at RV and $P_E$max at TLC are given in Table 3.1. $P_E$max values predicted by Black and Hyatt are considerably higher than those observed in many apparently normal subjects, hence it is reasonable to accept the lower limit of normal value for $P_E$max to be 100 cmH$_2$O for men and 80 cmH$_2$O for women, 20 years old and over.

Possible Problems

A result below normal for any techniques requiring maximal effort, for example, $P_I$max or $P_E$max, may be due to back pain or abdominal pain; inability to keep lips tightly sealed around the mouthpiece; less than maximum effort; or instructions poorly understood. Fatigue of respiratory muscle due to testing may also result in low readings. In such instances, the subject requires plenty of rest between efforts. If any of these factors contributed to a low reading, they should be noted on the report.

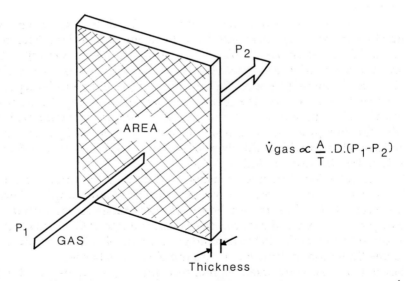

$$\dot{V}gas \propto \frac{A}{T} . D . (P_1 - P_2)$$

Figure 3.20 Diffusion of gas across the alveolar membrane. The volume of gas per unit time ($\dot{V}$gas) that diffuses across the membrane depends on the tissue area available for diffusion (A), the tissue thickness (T), the difference in gas partial pressure between the two sides (P_1-P_2). D = diffusion constant. (Modified from West J.B. Respiratory Physiology—the Essentials. Baltimore: WIlliams & Wilkins. With permission Williams & Wilkins © 1974.)

DIFFUSING CAPACITY (OR TRANSFER FACTOR) OF THE LUNG

The transfer of gas across the alveolar membrane occurs by diffusion. The diffusion of a gas depends upon the tissue area available for diffusion (A), the tissue thickness (T), the difference in gas partial pressure between the two sides $(P_1 - P_2)$ (Figure 3.20). The rate of transfer is also affected by a diffusion constant (D) which depends on the properties of the tissue and the specific gas. The constant is proportional to the solubility of the gas and inversely proportional to the square root of the molecular weight (MW).

$$\left(D \propto \frac{Sol}{\sqrt{MW}} \right)$$

All these factors are related by:

$$\dot{V}gas \propto \frac{A}{T} D(P_1 - P_2)$$

$\dot{V}$ = volume of gas per unit time. In this instance $\dot{V}$gas is the rate of flow (or diffusion) of the gas.

Measurement of the diffusing capacity of the lung is made whenever a diffusion problem is suspected. For example, in fibrosing alveolitis the diffusion is reduced due to thickening of the alveolar membrane. In emphysema the diffusion is reduced because the area for gas exchange is considerably diminished.

Carbon monoxide (CO) is used to measure the diffusing capacity of the lung since it has a very high affinity with haemoglobin (Hb). This means that, as CO moves across the blood–gas barrier into the blood cell, it binds with Hb allowing a large amount of CO to be taken up by the cell with almost no increase in partial pressure. This prevents any appreciable back pressure from developing so that the gas continues to move rapidly across the alveolar wall. Consequently, the transfer of CO into the blood is only limited by the diffusion properties of the blood–gas barrier and not by the amount of blood available, providing the Hb is within normal limits. The transfer of CO is said to be diffusion limited.

To measure the diffusing capacity of the lung for carbon monoxide (D_{LCO}), very low concentrations of CO are inspired and samples of expired gas are collected and measured. From the ratio of the CO concentrations in the inspired and expired gas, the disappearance rate of CO is calculated. If the concentration of CO in the expired gas is relatively high then there must be some limitation to diffusion across the blood–gas barrier.

Several methods are used to measure the D_{LCO}, however, the most commonly used is the *single breath method*. In this method the subject takes a single breath (from RV to TLC) of CO, air and helium mixture and breath holds for 10 seconds. The rate of disappearance of CO from the alveolar gas is calculated by measuring the inspired and expired concentrations of CO

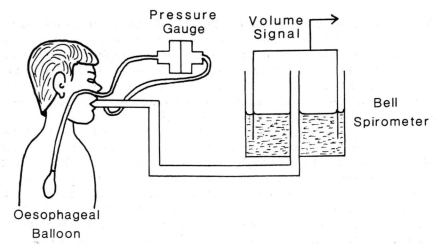

Figure 3.21   Diagrammatic representation of circuitry for the measurement of static compliance.

with an infrared analyser or gas chromatograph. Helium is inspired with the CO to measure the volume, that is, RV, which dilutes the CO. The transfer of CO can only be measured after taking this dilution into account. If the lung volume is reduced the D_{LCO} may appear low, however, it is possible that the lung units remaining have a normal diffusing capacity. D_{LCO} related to lung volume is called the transfer coefficient, K_{CO}:

$$K_{CO} = \frac{D_{LCO}}{V_A}$$

V_A = accessible gas volume

It is important to know the subject's Hb when measuring D_{LCO} since anaemia may result in a low D_{LCO} when the blood–gas barrier is normal.

Normal values for D_{LCO} are given in Crapo and Morris.[14] The measurement of D_{LCO} is usually done by trained laboratory personnel in specialized units.

COMPLIANCE AND ELASTIC RECOIL

Compliance of the lung is a measure of how distensible the lung is, that is, how easily it can be stretched. It is defined as the change in lung volume per unit pressure change across the lung. The pressure change across the lung is the transpulmonary pressure which is the difference between the pressure at the mouth and pleural pressure. To measure pleural pressure a small catheter with a thin-walled balloon surrounding its lower end is swallowed and positioned in the lower third of the oesophagus where pressure changes closely approximate pleural pressure changes (since this part of the oesophagus is in the thorax between the lung and the chest wall) (Figure 3.21).

The muscular force applied across the lung during inspiration is translated into changes in pleural pressure which stretch the lung and result in volume changes on inspiration. The greater the force applied, the more the lung is stretched and the bigger the volume change. This relationship between force and stretch or between pressure and volume is measured under static conditions and is known as *static compliance*. Static conditions means zero flow. The subject takes a big breath in to TLC and then breathes out to near RV, stopping at various intervals so that pressure and volume can be measured. The resultant normal pressure–volume curve looks like that in Figure 3.22. The relationship between pressure and volume is not linear, that is, there is no single value for compliance which applies over the entire vital capacity. Compliance is usually calculated by taking the best fitting line which applies over the tidal volume range in the vital capacity.

If the lungs are 'stiff', that is, less compliant or less easily stretched due to disease processes which cause fibrosis of the lung, a greater pressure is required to produce the same change in volume. This is because some of the elastic fibres have been replaced by collagen and fibrous tissue. If the lungs are 'floppy', that is, more compliant, as occurs in emphysema or with ageing, a smaller pressure change is required to produce the same change in volume. This is because elastic fibres have been lost without being replaced by collagen or fibrous tissue. Figure 3.22 shows the pressure–volume curves of decreased and increased compliance.

Compliance of the lung is dependent on lung size. A small adult lung will distend relatively less than a large adult lung of the same age if the same distending force is applied. This does not mean that the lungs of the small adult have different elasticity to the large adult, only that they are smaller. Both lungs may have much the same elastic properties when related to lung volume. In order to judge whether lung tissue has normal elastic properties both the compliance of the lung *and* the lung volume at which compliance is measured must be known. Compliance per unit lung volume is called *specific*

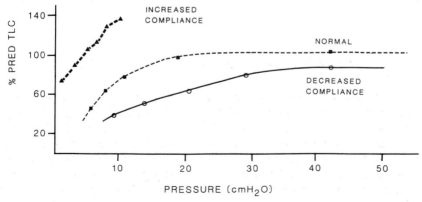

Figure 3.22 Normal pressure–volume curve compared with that of increased and decreased compliance.

compliance. Full details of the measurement of compliance are outside the scope of this chapter. For further details the reader is referred to Cotes.[15]

Other tests that are available in the pulmonary function laboratory and that can add valuable information to the investigation of lung disorders are:

(a) The measurement of arterial blood gases. For normal values see Table 3.1.
(b) The response of a subject to exercise in order to assess:
    (i) if the normal ventilatory reserves are preserved (see Chapter 7), or
    (ii) if exercise causes an increase in airway obstruction as occurs in exercise-induced asthma.
(c) Inhalation of substances such as mecholyl, histamine or hypertonic saline to assess if the airways are hyper-reactive as would be the case if the subject had asthma.

CONCLUSION

Although this chapter is not intended to be an exhaustive description of all pulmonary function tests, it is hoped that since the more commonly used tests are described in detail, the reader will have a better understanding of the value of such tests and will use this chapter as a guide when carrying them out. The ability to interpret pulmonary function tests enables the therapist better to understand the clinical condition of the patient and, as a consequence, plan the most appropriate intervention.

REFERENCES

1. Jones N.L., Campbell E.J.M., Edwards R.H.T., *et al*. (1982). *Clinical Exercise Testing*, 2nd edn. Philadelphia: W.B. Saunders, p. 245.
2. Grimby G., Soderholm B. (1963). Spirometric studies in normal subjects: III static lung volumes and maximum voluntary ventilation in adults with a note on physical fitness. *Acta Med. Scand.*, **173**, 199.
3. Polgar G., Promadhat V. (1971). *Pulmonary Function Testing in Children; Techniques and Standards*. Philadelphia: W.B. Saunders.
4. Hruby J., Butle J. (1975). Variability of routine pulmonary function tests. *Thorax*, **30**, 548.
5. Knudson R.J., Slatin R.C., Lebowitz M.D., *et al*. (1976). The maximal expiratory flow-volume curve: Normal standards, variability and effects of age. *Am. Rev. Respir. Dis.*, **113**, 587.
6. Ferris B.G., Anderson P.O., Zickmaniel R. (1968). Prediction values for screening tests of pulmonary function. *Am. Rev. Respir. Dis.* **91**, 252–261.
7. Gregg I., Nun A.J. (1973). Peak expiratory flow in normal subjects. *Br. Med. J.*, **3**, 282.
8. Godfrey S., Kamburoff P.L., Nairn J.R. (1970). Spirometry, lung volumes and airways resistance in normal children aged 5 to 18 years. *Br. J. Dis. Chest*, **64**, 15.

9. Friedman M., Walker S. (1975). Assessment of lung function using the airflow meter. *Lancet*, **1**, 310.
10. Crapo R.O., Morris A.H., Clayton P.D., *et al.* (1982). Lung volumes in healthy nonsmoking adults. *Bull. Europ. Physiopath. Resp.*, **18**, 419.
11. Clausen J.L., Zarins L.P. (1982). Estimation of lung volumes from chest radiographs. In *Pulmonary Function Testing. Guidelines and Controversies* (Clausen J.L., ed.). New York: Academic Press, pp. 155.
12. Wilson S.H., Cook N.T., Edwards R.H.T., *et al.* (1984). Predicted normal values for maximal respiratory mouth pressures in caucasian adults and children. *Thorax*, **39**, 535.
13. Black F., Hyatt R.E. (1961). Maximal respiratory pressures: Normal values and relationship to age and sex. *Am. Rev. Respir. Dis.* **99**, 696.
14. Crapo R.O., Morris A.H. (1981). Standardized single breath normal values for carbon monoxide diffusing capacity. *Am. Rev. Respir. Dis.*, **123**, 185.
15. Cotes J.E. (1975). *Lung Function*, 3rd edn. Oxford: Blackwell Scientific Publications.
16. Crapo R.O., Morris A.H., Gardner R.M. (1981). Reference spirometric values using techniques and equipment that meet ATS recommendations. *Am. Rev. Respir. Dis.*, **123**, 659.
17. Mellemgaard K. (1966). The alveolar-arterial oxygen difference: Its size and components in normal man. *Acta Physiol. Scand.*, **67**, 10.
18. Turino G.M. (Chairman). (1977). Conference report: Workshop on assessment of respiratory control in humans: VII. Measurements of the responsiveness of the respiratory apparatus in disease. *Am. Rev. Respir. Dis.*, **115**, 883.

FURTHER READING

West J.B. (1985) *Respiratory Physiology—the Essentials*, 3rd edn. Baltimore: Williams & Wilkins.

West J.B. (1987). *Pulmonary Pathophysiology—the Essentials*, 3rd edn. Baltimore: Williams & Wilkins.

Comroe J.H. (1974) *Physiology of Respiration*, 2nd edn. Chicago: Year Book Medical Publishers.

Clausen J.C., ed. (1982). *Pulmonary Function Testing. Guidelines and Controversies*. New York: Academic Press.

Chapter 4

Chest Radiology

MARGARET STEWART

INTRODUCTION

By far the majority of radiological examinations undertaken in any hospital are the relatively cheap and easily performed chest radiographs which provide a wealth of information in the assessment of both the medical and surgical patient. Correct interpretation of any chest film, however, requires a familiarity with the normal anatomical appearance and an understanding of the technical aspects.

STANDARD RADIOGRAPHIC TECHNIQUE

For the standard postero-anterior (PA) view, the cassette containing the X-ray film is placed in front of the patient, against the chest. The X-ray tube is 2.0 metres behind the patient so that during the exposure the beam travels from behind the patient through to the film, anterior to the patient. Mobile X-rays or those done on patients unable to stand are usually anteroposterior (AP) views when the cassette is propped up behind the sitting or lying patient and the X-ray beam travels from in front of the patient through to the film. For screening examinations in patients under 40 years a PA view alone is usually sufficient but in older patients, or in those with known or suspected abnormalities, then a lateral view is also necessary. The left lateral view is usually performed, i.e. the left side of the patient is closest to the X-ray film. This is because more of the left lung is usually obscured by the heart on the PA view and the left lateral view allows slightly better definition of the structures closest to the film. If the PA view shows an abnormality in the right lung, then a right lateral view may provide more information.

The film should be exposed on *full inspiration*, i.e. at total lung volume, so that the lower halves of the lungs are better seen and the costophrenic angles and the heart are sharply delineated. These areas are not well seen on expiratory views, which may lead to over-diagnosis of pathology. With a good inspiration, approximately 10 posterior, horizontal ribs or 6 anterior, more vertical ribs should be visible.

56

The *exposure time* is as short as possible to minimize movement blur of the heart, lungs and diaphragm. Correct exposure of the film allows for the size of the patient and, to some degree, the underlying pulmonary pathology so that patients with dense lungs due to pneumonia or oedema will need a greater exposure than patients with relatively destroyed lungs from emphysema or those who have had previous surgery. Too great an exposure results in a 'blacker' film so that small abnormalities are almost impossible to detect and too small an exposure results in a 'whiter' film due to poor penetration of the patient. This may result in over-diagnosing pathology in the white lungs but missing mediastinal lesions because of the lack of relevant detail. Exposures of subsequent chest examinations should be as constant as possible to allow comparison of serial films.

It is important that the patient is *correctly positioned* as the X-ray film can be quite misleading if the patient is not straight at the time of exposure. This is obviously vital with the AP view in the postoperative or intensive care patient. Correct positioning of the patient can be judged by measuring the distance from the medial end of the clavicle to the central thoracic spine. When the distance on either side is the same then the patient is straight, but if the patient is rotated then the clavicle/spine distances will no longer be equal. If the patient's right side is away from the film, then right-sided mediastinal structures become more prominent and the right lung appears 'blacker' than the left. If the left side of the body is away from the film, then the left lung may appear more radiolucent or 'blacker' and the right lung 'whiter' or less radiolucent. The left hilum also appears smaller as it is hidden by the heart. If a difference in lung density is seen then the patient's position should always be checked before other causes of altered lung density such as pneumothorax, previous mastectomy or pneumonia are considered.

In summary, accurate assessment of the chest film is aided by a correctly exposed film of a properly positioned patient who has taken a large inspiration.

NORMAL ANATOMY

The normal anatomy of a *postero-anterior* radiograph is seen in Figure 4.1. The trachea is essentially a midline structure, although slight deviation to the right after entering the thorax at the level of the clavicles is a normal finding and should not be misinterpreted as evidence of displacement. The tracheal walls are parallel except on the left side where just above the carina a smooth indentation is caused by the aortic arch. Calcification of the tracheal cartilage rings is not an uncommon finding, especially in the older patient. The trachea divides into right and left major bronchi at the carina. The angle of bifurcation is variable but the right main bronchus is seen as straighter and more vertical than the left. The azygos vein and azygos node are seen as a short convex shadow in the right tracheobronchial angle. The vertical

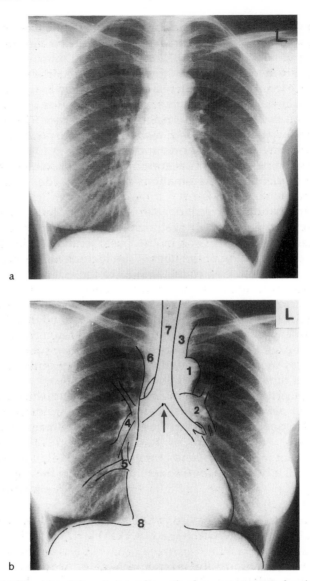

Figure 4.1 *(a) Normal postero-anterior radiograph of an asymptomatic female. (b) The normal structures are outlined and numbered: 1, Aorta; 2, Left pulmonary artery; 3, Left subclavian artery; 4, Right pulmonary artery; 5, Right lower lobe pulmonary veins; 6, Superior vena cava; 7, Trachea. The arrow points to the carina.*

shadow of the right side of the mediastinum, below the medial end of the clavicle, is the right lateral margin of the superior vena cava, which runs between the first and third anterior costal cartilages.

On the left side of the superior mediastinum is the curve of the subclavian vessels over the apex of the lung. Below this is one of the landmarks of the mediastinum – the convexity of the aortic arch. Between this and the next convexity of the left pulmonary artery is the shallow area called the aortopulmonary window.

The pulmonary hila are usually of equal density. However, the left is higher than the right because the left pulmonary artery curves up and over and then down behind the left main bronchus, while the right pulmonary artery lies at the same level as the right main bronchus. This pulmonary artery bifurcates in the hilum, which results in the normal angular appearance of the right hilum.

The clavicles should be horizontal and the scapulae should be as far lateral as possible to allow clear assessment of the lung fields. The lungs are normally of equal density with the typical pattern of branching vessels extending out towards the periphery. The diaphragm should be seen as a sharp outline except medially where the cardiophrenic fat pads are situated. The costophrenic angles laterally should be seen as acute. The right hemidiaphragm is usually higher than the left by approximately half an interspace or 1–2 cm.

The size of the heart is usually estimated by comparing the widest diameter of the heart to the diameter of the thorax at the level of insertion of the diaphragm. If the heart size is less than half this diameter then it is judged to be of normal size whereas if it is greater than half this size then the heart is judged to be enlarged. Any heart, however, whose transverse diameter is greater than 15.5–16 cm is considered enlarged, no matter what the diameter of the chest.

Most of the markings seen on a normal chest film are due to the density of the blood-filled pulmonary arteries and veins. The pulmonary arteries, carrying the deoxygenated blood to the lungs, are the main vessels of the hilar regions. The pulmonary veins returning the oxygenated blood to the heart are best seen at the lung bases running horizontally towards the left atrium but may also be seen lying lateral to the arteries in the upper lobes. As the heart largely obscures the left lower zone, this differentiation is better appreciated in the right lung.

Under normal conditions in an erect individual, blood flow is not evenly distributed in the lungs but occurs predominantly through the lung bases with relative under-perfusion of the upper zones. Consequently, the blood vessels to the bases are normally larger than those to the upper zones. If the patient is supine, this blood flow differential is lost and the upper lobe vessels may be seen to be as large as, or even larger than, the lower lobe vessels. This may result in an erroneous diagnosis of cardiac failure.

The normal anatomy of a *lateral* chest radiograph is seen in Figure 4.2. The tracheal air column is situated centrally within the superior mediastinum. Anterior to it is seen a roughly rectangular area of density due to the shadow of the great vessels and posteriorly there is the shadow of the posterior aortic arch, the superior curving margin of which is usually easily identified. As the aortic arch is prominent in both PA and lateral projections, a small lung lesion can be accurately localized by correlating its position in relation to the

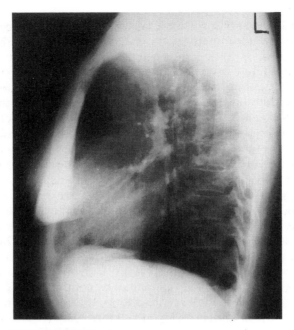

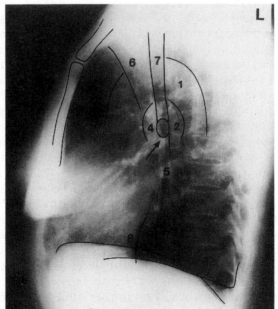

Figure 4.2   (a) Normal lateral radiograph of an asymptomatic female. (b) The normal structures are outlined and numbered: 1, Aorta; 2, Left pulmonary artery; 4, Right pulmonary artery; 5, Confluence of the pulmonary veins; 6, Brachiocephalic vessels; 7, Trachea; 8, Inferior vena cava. The arrow points to the orifice of the left main bronchus.

arch on the two views. The retrosternal area above the heart only contains a little fat in the adult and is, therefore, radiolucent but in the child this is the site of the thymus gland causing a normal increase in density here.

In the middle of the chest, at the level of the hila, a black circular lucency in the line of the tracheal air column usually represents the left upper lobe bronchus. Anteriorly lies the curved density of the right pulmonary artery and posteriorly lies another density, the left pulmonary artery. Immediately inferiorly lies the apparent tangle of pulmonary veins. Calcification of the heart valves, if present, is also better appreciated on the lateral view.

The scapulae and axillary soft tissue overlie the upper thoracic vertebrae and the posterior portions of the lung fields making these areas appear quite dense. Alternatively, below this level down to the diaphragm the thoracic vertebrae should be quite clearly outlined as they are surrounded by the normal air-filled lungs. Any change from this arrangement with an increase in density obscuring the lower vertebrae should raise the possibility of an abnormality in the lower lobes such as collapse or consolidation. The diaphragm should be sharply outlined, except anteriorly on the left where the heart is situated. The posterior costophrenic angles should also be acute.

A working knowledge of the normal bronchial anatomy is fundamental in interpreting chest films. Once an abnormality is detected, accurate placement may help in the diagnosis, for example, tuberculous opacities are usually in the apical and posterior segments of the upper lobes and superior segments of the lower lobes, whereas hydatid cysts are more common in the right lower lobe. Physiotherapy, so necessary in the treatment of pneumonias and for postoperative patients, can be better directed and so much more effective if the location of the consolidation or collapse is known. In addition, bronchoscopy and transbronchial biopsy are more likely to yield a positive result if the physician can accurately aim for the segment containing the abnormality.

The *pulmonary fissures* are the pleural divisions of the lobes of the lungs. The oblique or major fissures are well seen on the lateral view and separate the upper and middle lobes from the lower lobe on the right and the upper lobe, which includes the lingula, from the lower lobe on the left. The oblique fissures run forwards and inferiorly from approximately the lower border of the 4th thoracic vertebral body to meet the diaphragm 2–3 cm posterior to the cardiophrenic angle on either side, the left oblique fissure lying slightly posterior to the right. As the fissures undulate slightly they are not always seen in their entirety throughout the lungs and often only their lower portions are appreciated.

The horizontal fissure separates the upper from the middle lobe on the right. It is not usually present in the left lung. The fissure is well seen in both views of the chest radiograph, extending as a straight line from the mid-hilum laterally to the chest wall on the PA view and anteriorly to the sternum on the lateral view.

The superior or apical segment of either lower lobe lies immediately below the postero-superior portion of the oblique fissure but is above the level of the horizontal fissure. Any lesion, therefore, that lies in the perihilar area on the PA view above the level of the horizontal fissure may lie in either the upper lobe, anterior to the hilum, or in the apical segment of the lower lobe, posterior to the hilum. Such a difference in position requires widely different approaches for a possible biopsy and emphasizes the need for simultaneous evaluation of the fissures in both PA and lateral views in respect to any possible abnormality.

Abnormal disease states are reflected on the chest films by either an increase in radiographic density or by decreased radiographic density. There are numerous causes of both such abnormalities and it should be remembered that the final assessment of the particular radiographic abnormality should take into account the patient's history and physical examination as well as laboratory and pulmonary function test results. Diagnostic accuracy is improved considerably by correlation of the clinical and radiological findings.

INCREASED RADIOGRAPHIC DENSITY

The most common causes of an abnormal increase in density on the chest film would be pulmonary consolidation, lobar or segmental collapse, pleural effusion or neoplasm.

Consolidation

The density of consolidation is seen because fluid, pus, blood or abnormal cells have filled the alveoli, making them airless. Thus the term 'consolidation' as used by the radiologist is relatively non-specific as to the particular pathological process and refers to the pattern that may be seen most commonly with acute pneumonia and with pulmonary oedema but also with pulmonary infarction or contusion, as well as lymphoma or alveolar-cell carcinoma. Because the alveoli become filled with the pathological process at random and at different rates, consolidation initially may be incomplete, resulting in ill-defined or patchy densities with intervening areas of normal lung (Figure 4.3). As the condition progresses and more acinar air is replaced then the radiographic density increases and spreads within the lobe, perhaps eventually to be limited by the fissures as lobar consolidation. As the consolidation becomes more dense, the difference between the air-filled bronchi and the adjacent consolidated lung becomes more apparent and 'air-bronchograms' are seen (Figure 4.4). This is most common with consolidation due to acute infection or pulmonary oedema.

Some cases of pneumonia will show only a mild increase in pulmonary markings or areas of minor consolidation, a pattern common to the viral pneumonias. Other pneumonias may be very extensive, involving multiple

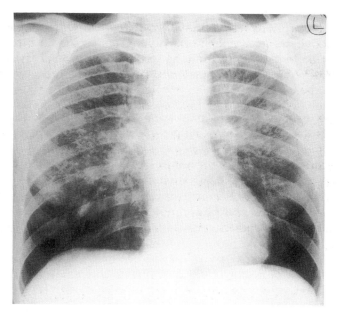

Figure 4.3   The patchy, poorly-defined pattern of pulmonary consolidation is seen bilaterally but is worse in the upper zones in this patient with pneumocystis pneumonia.

lobes, either uni- or bilaterally (the so-called 'double' pneumonia). Resolution of pneumonia usually takes two to three weeks but follows no definite radiological pattern.

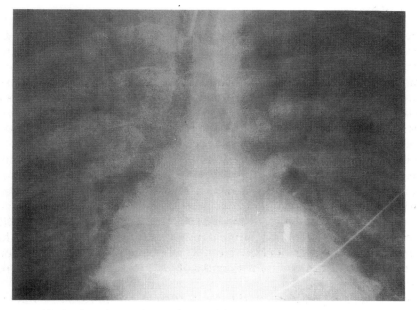

Figure 4.4   The 'air-bronchogram' sign – the consolidation is so dense in both lungs that the air-filled central bronchi stand out in stark relief.

As the pattern of consolidation in acute pneumonia is usually non-specific, no definite bacteriological aetiology can be inferred from the film alone. In the correct clinical setting, however, one of several organisms may cause a more characteristic pattern so that the appropriate microbiology tests may be performed.

1 Staphylococcal pneumonia may appear as multiple, rounded areas of consolidation which often cavitate and, in children, large air cysts or pneumatoceles may be a feature.
2 Klebsiella pneumonia may result in lobar consolidation that bulges the fissures and commonly causes cavitation.
3 Acute tuberculous pneumonia appears as soft, fluffy consolidation, usually in the apical and posterior segments of the upper and superior segments of the lower lobes and is commonly bilateral. Cavitation is a hallmark of active pathology. As pulmonary tuberculosis is a disease characterized by relapses and remissions, acute infection may be seen with evidence of healing from previous episodes. Fibrosis is then present, again most obvious in the upper lobes and often severe enough to cause deviation of the trachea. Calcifications, small and grouped in clusters, are common in the fibrotic areas.
4 Pneumocystis pneumonia usually occurs in patients who are immuno-suppressed because of corticosteroid therapy, organ transplantation, leukaemia or lymphoma, or the acquired immunodeficiency syndrome (AIDS). Early in the disease only a minor increase in density in the perihilar areas may be apparent but later dense bilateral air-space consolidation may be quite diffuse, mimicking pulmonary oedema. The lungs may appear to be very solid and the radiological changes often persist after clinical improvement begins.

Communication of an area of necrotic lung with the bronchial tree with subsequent expectoration results in an *abscess* cavity. Such cavities may vary in size from being only a centimetre in diameter to occupying an entire lobe. The wall of an acute abscess is thick and it may be nodular or smooth but an air–fluid level clearly makes the diagnosis (Figure 4.5). When an abscess develops in an acute infection, involvement of the pleural space may lead to the development of an empyema, occasionally with a broncho-pleural fistula. Resolution of the abscess over time may result in complete healing or may leave residual scarring, fibrosis or bronchiectasis.

Pulmonary consolidation does not of itself result in significant loss of volume of the lobe or lung, consequently the fissures, hila and diaphragm are usually in relatively normal position. If evidence of lobar collapse is present as well as the consolidation, then an underlying malignant cause should be suspected. Other confirmatory signs of malignancy should be looked for on the radiograph, such as an enlarged hilum, elevation of a hemidiaphragm because of phrenic nerve involvement or rib metastases.

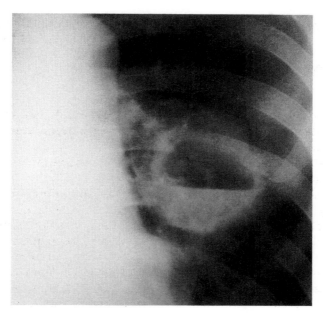

Figure 4.5   A close-up view of the left lung shows a large abscess cavity with a thick wall and an air–fluid level.

The group of interstitial lung diseases which includes sarcoidosis, idiopathic and drug-induced pulmonary fibrosis and eosinophilic granuloma presents quite a different radiographic appearance to pulmonary consolidation. In these conditions myriad small nodules are seen, usually with a reticular or 'lace-like' pattern throughout the lung fields. Often the radiograph shows only poorly expanded lungs, reflecting the reduction in lung volumes especially common with advanced interstitial fibrosis.

Collapse

If an airway is blocked by neoplasm, foreign body or mucus plugs then the air distal to the obstruction is absorbed and the affected lung collapses. The magnitude of the collapse and, therefore, the degree of radiological abnormality depends upon the size of the blocked airway. If a large central bronchus is obstructed, then total lobar collapse will be the result. Each lobe collapses towards the hilum in a characteristic pattern and the remainder of the lung expands to fill the vacated space. The consequent change from the normal anatomy with the shift of the fissures and the blood vessels leads to the radiological diagnosis of collapse.

Increase in density of the collapsed lobe is not always apparent, often not until a considerable volume loss has occurred but if there is coexisting consolidation within the collapsed lobe, then the increased radio-density of the lobe makes the diagnosis easier.

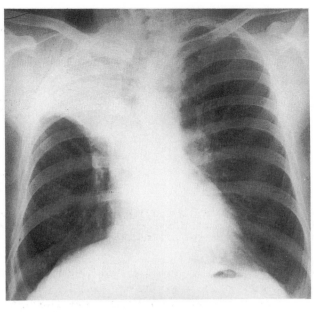

a

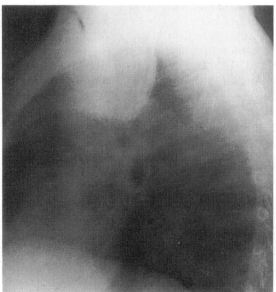

b

Figure 4.6   Collapse of the right upper lobe is seen in the PA projection (a) and lateral projection (b). The collapsed lobe is contiguous with the mediastinum in (a) so that no air shadow separates them. The inferior border is the upward curving horizontal fissure in both (a) and (b) and the posterior border in (b) is the anteriorly displaced upper half of the right oblique fissure. Rib crowding and tracheal shift are obvious. The patient had a central bronchial carcinoma.

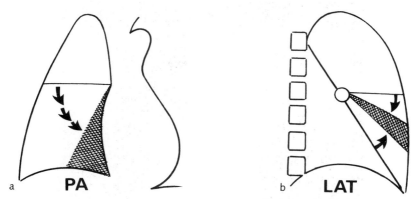

Figure 4.7   Diagrammatic representation of middle lobe collapse is seen in the PA projection (a) and lateral projection (b). Loss of the outline of the heart border on the PA view is characteristic of the collapse which is usually easily confirmed on the lateral view.

Right upper lobe collapse (Figure 4.6). The horizontal fissure moves upward, both on the PA and lateral views, and the superior part of the oblique fissure moves forward on the lateral view. The right hilum is elevated while the lower vessels of the hilum swing outwards. The trachea may deviate towards the collapse and there may occasionally be crowding of the upper right ribs.

Middle lobe collapse (Figure 4.7). There is downward displacement of the horizontal fissure with minimal upward movement of the lower oblique fissure. On the PA view the right cardiac border is usually obscured by the density of the adjacent collapsed lobe, that is, there is loss of the silhouette of the heart outline. The diagnosis is usually easier to make on the lateral rather than the PA view.

Left upper lobe collapse (Figure 4.8). There is usually increased opacity in the area of the left upper lobe and on the lateral view the oblique fissure is seen to be displaced well forwards. The left hilar vessels can no longer be distinguished, although there may be vascular markings present which are seen through the density. These are the blood vessels of the left lower lobe that grossly overexpand to occupy the space vacated by the collapsed upper lobe. Tracheal shift to the left is often present and rib crowding is occasionally seen. Because the lingula is part of the left upper lobe, there is no definite demarcation of the lower border in the left lung and the opacity of the upper lobar collapse fades inferiorly.

Lower lobe collapse (Figure 4.9). Due to a transient decrease in diaphragm function and mucus retention with poor inspiration, lower lobe collapse is a frequent occurrence in the postoperative patient when it usually involves several of the lower lobe segments and is frequently bilateral. Radiologically, lower lobe collapse is diagnosed on the lateral view by backward shift of the oblique fissure with increased density of the collapsed lobe overlying

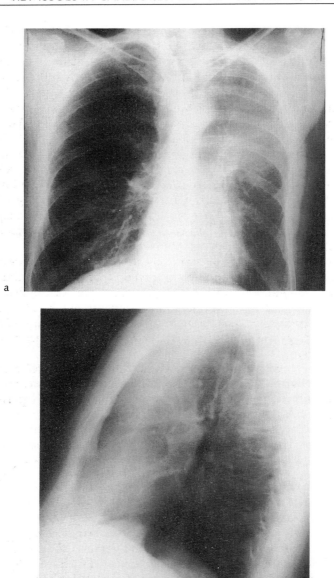

Figure 4.8   Left upper lobe collapse is present on the PA projection (a) and lateral projection (b). The outline of the aortic arch is seen on (a) as this is posterior to the collapse on (b) and outlined by the air-filled lower lobe. As there is no horizontal fissure there is no definite inferior margin to the density. Bronchoscopy revealed a left upper lobe carcinoma.

the lower thoracic vertebrae and loss of the outline of the posterior hemi-diaghram on the affected side. On the PA view, the density of the collapsed lobe is seen behind the heart, adjacent to the vertebral column on the left and behind the heart and in the cardiophrenic area on the right. Lower lobe collapse usually causes downward displacement of the superior hilar vessels and minor downward shift of the horizontal fissure accompanies right lower lobe collapse. The diaphragm may be displaced upwards but tracheal shift and rib crowding are not features.

Previous infections, thoracic surgery or pleural disease may cause distortion of the above 'classical' patterns of collapse. Pulmonary collapse is probably the most common sign of bronchogenic carcinoma and it may be segmental, lobar or massive, involving an entire lung. Amongst hospital patients, especially those after recent surgery, lower lobe collapse is a common radiological finding and usually responds well to physiotherapy (Figure 4.10).

Collapse of a lobe or lobar segments may also be the result of scarring and fibrosis due to previous radiotherapy or infection, particularly tuberculosis. In such cases, the signs of collapse, in particular shift of the fissures and crowding of the vessels are present, usually with streaky bands of fibrosis, but there is no evidence of consolidation. These areas of collapsed lung are often longstanding and unchanged on serial films taken over a period of months or years.

Small areas of basal subsegmental collapse, often seen as 'band shadows' in the lower lobes and usually associated with small effusions, may be the only radiological evidence of pulmonary emboli, although peripherally placed areas of consolidation also occur.

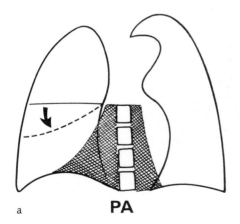
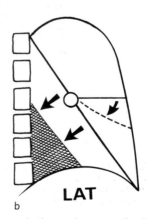

a   **PA**   b   **LAT**

Figure 4.9 Diagrammatic representation of lower lobe collapse – both are drawn on the PA projection (a) and the lateral projection (b). Both the left and right lower lobes have a similar appearance on the lateral view when collapsed, with increased density seen postero-inferiorly obscuring the costophrenic gutter and ipsilateral posterior hemidiaphragm. On the PA view the collapsed lobe is seen adjacent to the vertebral column, in the cardiophrenic area on the right and behind the heart on the left.

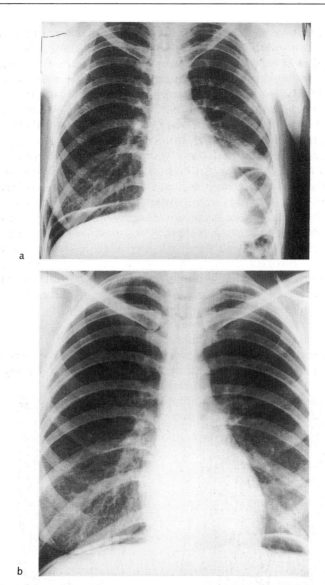

a

b

Figure 4.10   Left lower lobe collapse (a) and re-expansion of the lobe after physiotherapy (b). The density of the collapsed lobe clears completely and the diaphragm returns to its normal position after treatment. The collapse was due to retained secretions after a recent abdominal operation. Note the subdiaphragmatic air.

Pleural Effusion

Pleural fluid is formed and absorbed constantly and any abnormality of the normal metabolic pathway results in accumulation of fluid in the pleural cavity, seen as the homogeneous opacity of a pleural effusion. Usually, pleural fluid will accumulate in the most dependent areas, that is, around the lung bases in an erect patient where it first fills the posterior costophrenic angles, extending medially and upwards into the fissures obscuring and compressing the underlying lung (Figure 4.11). If the patient is supine, then the fluid layers posteriorly in the dependent area and the whole lung field will appear relatively more dense than that on the normal side. Lung markings should be seen through the effusion in their normal position unless there is coexistent lung pathology. Occasionally pleural effusions are large enough to 'white-out' entirely a hemithorax so that no features of the underlying lung can be distinguished. In such cases with a massive effusion, the heart and mediastinum are shifted to the opposite side unless there is tethering of the mediastinum by malignant involvement of central nodes.

Smaller effusions may be loculated in unusual collections because of pleural adhesions in fissures or in the subpulmonary position between the lung and the diaphragm. Such loculated effusions may often cause confusing shadows and may be erroneously diagnosed as lung tumours. Recently ultrasound has become a useful non-invasive way of accurately assessing loculated collections of pleural fluid and catheter drainage of empyemas using ultrasound control is becoming an established technique.

Neoplasm

Pulmonary masses are most often bronchial carcinomas, especially in males over 40 years. The differential diagnosis includes, among others,

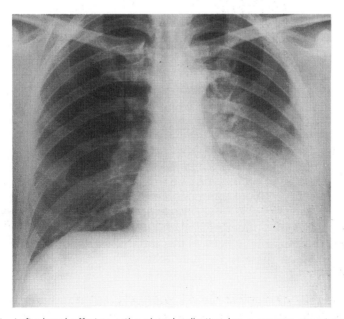

Figure 4.11   Left pleural effusion – the pleural collection has a concave superior margin and obliterates the outline of the underlying hemidiaphragm. This effusion was secondary to a lower lobe pneumonia.

tuberculoma or hamartoma in smaller nodules and abscess and lymphoma in larger masses and, of course, metastases especially if the lesions are multiple. A malignant tumour tends to have ill-defined or lobulated margins but may be of any size and in any part of the lung. Cavitation is not uncommon but calcification in a carcinoma is exceedingly rare and, if present in a mass indicates that the lesion is more likely to be benign than malignant. Most pulmonary masses are now also evaluated with computerized axial tomography.

DECREASED RADIOGRAPHIC DENSITY

A decrease in lung density may be localized as with a lung cyst or may be the result of generalized destruction of pulmonary parenchyma as with emphysema. It may also be due to deflation of the lung because of the presence of a pneumothorax.

Lung Cysts

The majority of cysts in the lung itself are acquired, usually as the result of infection. There remains a small number which may be of congenital origin and it is impossible to differentiate between the two varieties on the radiological appearances alone. Cysts may be air or fluid filled and when air filled are often large with a smooth thin wall.

Emphysema

This chronic disease entity presumes some destruction of the underlying lung which is reflected on the plain chest film as a generalized decrease in the size and number of peripheral markings resulting in increased blackness of the lungs. Air trapping due to the associated chronic obstructive pathology results in an increase in volume of the lungs seen on the radiograph as an increase in the AP diameter of the chest, often resulting in outward bowing of the sternum, flattening of the diaphragm and a long narrow heart. Emphysematous bullae, rounded radiolucencies of varying size usually in the upper zones, confirm the diagnosis when present.

Unilateral emphysema may be due to a localized obstruction such as an inhaled foreign body, most commonly in children. Because of the ball-valve obstruction allowing air to enter the lung but preventing expiration, the affected lung becomes hyperinflated and does not reduce in size as it should on expiration. Comparison films in inspiration and expiration usually show the air trapping on the affected side with shift of the mediastinum to the normal side.

Pneumothorax

Air in the pleural cavity results in the formation of a pneumothorax, seen as a lucent gas space devoid of pulmonary vessels between the chest wall and

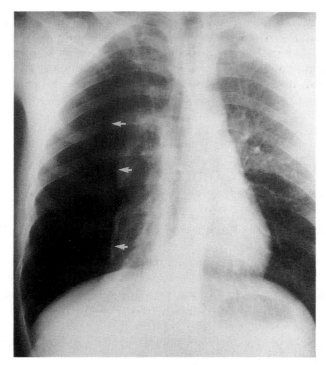

Figure 4.12   A large right pneumothorax is present with collapse of the underlying lung, the edge of which is arrowed. There is shift of the heart and mediastinum away from the affected side.

the outer margin of the lung. By far the most common cause of a pneumothorax is spontaneous rupture of an air bleb, usually in young healthy males in whom the pneumothorax is often recurrent and frequently bilateral.

Other causes, however, include chronic obstructive pulmonary disease, usually in the older age group, where the development of a pneumothorax may be the cause of sudden clinical deterioration. Any chronic interstitial lung disease such as sarcoidosis, histiocytosis and pulmonary fibrosis, is more prone to pneumothorax, as are malignant neoplasms and lung abscesses.

Traumatic causes of pneumothorax include chest operations, rib fractures, barotrauma from mechanical ventilation and as a result of invasive procedures, such as lung biopsy and central line placement.

Pneumothoraces are best seen on the PA view (Figure 4.12) and a film taken in expiration may show the pneumothorax better than the usual inspiratory view. Care must be taken not to confuse artefacts such as skin or bandage folds overlying the lung for the edge of the displaced lung, particularly on AP films taken in bed. Accurate estimation of the size of a pneumothorax is very difficult and percentage estimations generally underestimate the true size. It is usually best to relate the lung edge to the nearest posterior rib.

If there is a pleural flap present, air may continually expand the pleural space resulting in the formation of a tension pneumothorax, diagnosed by shift of the mediastinum away from the side of the pneumothorax, depression of the hemidiaphragm and expansion of the ribs on the affected side. The presence of air under tension compresses the lung and decreases venous return to the heart and may rapidly lead to a life-threatening emergency.

CARDIAC FAILURE

Left ventricular failure is one of the most commonly encountered conditions in clinical practice (Figure 4.13). Although there are many precipitating causes, the most common of which is ischaemic heart disease, the radiological appearances are usually diagnostic. The heart is usually enlarged. The earliest sign of cardiac failure in the lungs may be quite subtle with shift of the blood flow to the upper lobe vessels causing distension of these vessels. This phase of pulmonary venous hypertension may be followed by interstitial pulmonary oedema when fluid escapes into the interstitial tissues and is characterized by Kerley 'B' lines, which are short lines arranged in stepladder fashion along the lower lung margins. If the heart continues to fail

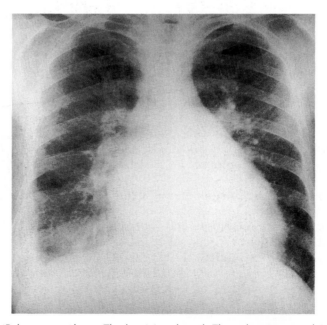

Figure 4.13 Pulmonary oedema. The heart is enlarged. The pulmonary vessels are distended especially in the upper lobes and increased markings are seen in the lung fields with early consolidation in the right lower lobe. Note the small right effusion.

then alveolar oedema develops with overflow of fluid into the alveolae, reflected by an increase in 'greyness' of the lungs or in worse cases with pulmonary consolidation that may be diffuse or may be localized to the basal areas or occasionally in the perihilar regions as 'bats wing' oedema. Pulmonary oedema is usually accompanied by small pleural effusions and characteristically may appear and clear relatively quickly as cardiac compensation is restored.

Not all cases of pulmonary oedema are due to cardiac failure. Renal failure, intravenous fluid overload, drug abuse, neurosurgical events and the adult respiratory distress syndrome may all result in pulmonary oedema. Despite the varying causes the radiological picture remains similar remembering, however, that consolidation due to pulmonary oedema also has to be differentiated from consolidation due to other causes, especially lobar pneumonia.

Right ventricular failure or cor pulmonale (Figure 4.14) is the result of end-stage chronic lung disease or recurrent pulmonary emboli. Radiologically the changes of the underlying pulmonary problem will often be seen. The heart enlarges as does the right ventricle and the central pulmonary arteries are enlarged. The peripheral pulmonary arteries are diminished.

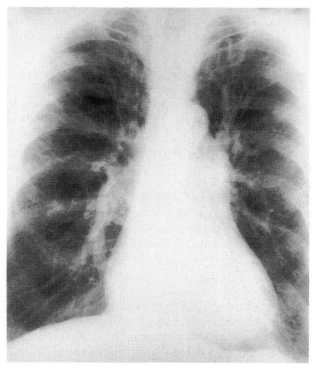

Figure 4.14   Cor pulmonale. Note that the heart is enlarged and the right ventricle, pulmonary trunk and central pulmonary arteries are prominent. The peripheral lung fields show no obvious abnormality.

The diagnosis is assisted by electrocardiogram findings and clinical features. Again abnormal appearances are exaggerated during acute exacerbations and may rapidly improve with improvement in the clinical condition.

COMPUTERIZED TOMOGRAPHY

Thoracic computerized tomography (CT) has become a valuable supplementary examination to the plain chest radiograph. The patient has to lie supine within a circular gantry containing the X-ray tube. During an exposure a narrow X-ray beam scans across the thorax passing through to detectors on the other side. The intensity of the emergent photons is transmitted electronically to a computer which can then print out the tissue densities and reconstruct an image of the scanned area. The patient is then moved through the scanner, usually at 1 cm intervals, and the scan is repeated at each stop, so that for a CT examination of the chest there are approximately 25–30 images to be examined in sequence.

Computerized tomographic scanning has been quickly adopted into clinical medicine because of three main advantages. First, the ability of CT to show the chest in transverse section, thus eliminating the superimposition of major structures. This has had a major impact in evaluation of the mediastinum and in the accurate localization of possible abnormalities. Secondly, the ability to detect small differences in tissue density, usually presented on a scale of Hounsfield units (HU), named after Geoffrey Hounsfield, the inventor of CT. The scale ranges about the standard of water at 0 HU so that the ribs and bones are seen as very white because of their high density and the lungs appear black because of their low air density. Cystic lesions have densities 0 to +10 HU while soft-tissue masses are usually in the +30 to +50 range. Hence, an abnormality on the CT scan can be characterized as to its likely tissue density so that the usually benign cystic or fatty lesions can be differentiated from the more probably malignant soft-tissue masses.

The third major advantage of CT is that all structures at one level can be simultaneously evaluated. For each X-ray exposure, just by adjusting the contrast of the picture, the area in question can be evaluated with regard to the lungs, the mediastinum or the bones. This eliminates multiple examinations such as oblique rib views, whole lung tomography or barium swallows.

CT has been found to be invaluable in the work-up of the patient with an abnormality suspected on the plain chest film when it is often difficult to be certain whether an abnormality is indeed present or whether the suspected abnormality is truly pathological. Unfortunately, there is as yet no foolproof way to distinguish between benign and malignant masses on CT alone. Nevertheless, CT can accurately localize the lesion, especially if it is small, better directing the subsequent biopsy procedure either by percutaneous needle or via the bronchoscope.

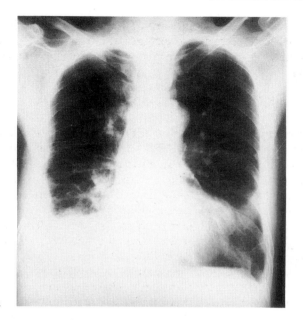

a

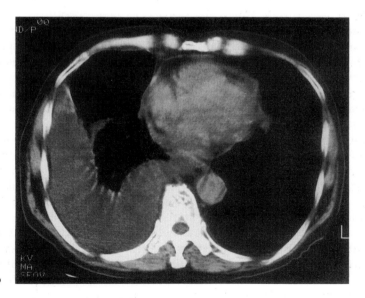

b

Figure 4.15   Plain chest film (a) showing increased density at the right base. CT scans of this area on mediastinal settings (b) show that the density is a large pleural effusion. Scan (c) shows the compression of the underlying lung with bands of collapse between the effusion and the heart. The left lung is clear. The patient had a malignant pleural effusion.

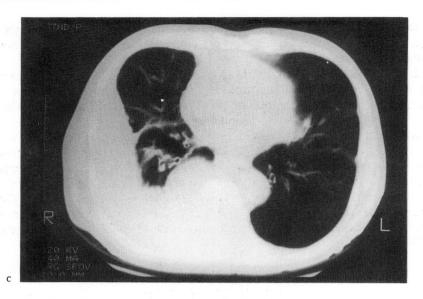

c

Estimation of the extent of tumour, either carcinoma or lymphoma, is crucial for accurate staging and prognosis and is the basis of many clinical decisions by the thoracic surgeons, radiotherapists and oncologists. Thus, the scans are evaluated for mediastinal or hilar lymphadenopathy, evidence of mediastinal invasion, pleural or pericardial effusions, as well as assessing the lung fields for small secondary deposits. To assess the liver and adrenal glands for metastases, the scans are easily continued into the upper abdomen.

If major surgery is planned, then it is important to exclude metastatic lung nodules. CT can show nodules as small as 3 mm diameter, whereas plain chest films show nodules 8–10 mm in size.

CT is useful for evaluation of pleural disease (Figure 4.15) especially in differentiation of lung abscess from empyema, and in the assessment of malignant mesotheliomas of the pleura.

CT, however, does have its limitations. The patient has to be able to lie still and hold their breath during the examination which is mildly invasive in that intravenous iodinated contrast is usually given to enhance the vessels allowing differentiation from the surrounding soft tissues. The scans are also relatively expensive. It is not useful in cases of consolidation, such as uncomplicated pneumonia, nor is it necessary with minor atelectasis. Its role in pulmonary fibrosis and bronchiectasis is still being assessed and not all the nodules or nodes that CT shows are pathological.

MAGNETIC RESONANCE IMAGING (MRI)

This lately developed, highly technical imaging modality uses radio-waves modified by a strong magnetic field to produce a diagnostic image. It uses no

X-rays but results in an image very similar to the CT cross-sectional image. It can also image the chest in multiple planes so that coronal and sagittal scans are easily performed.

MRI has established itself in the imaging of the brain and spinal cord but so far has had only a minor role in chest imaging, mainly confined to evaluation of cardiac and great vessel abnormalities and, to a lesser extent, the evaluation of mediastinal masses.

MRI is very expensive and produces images of the chest no better than a good quality CT scan. It also takes longer to perform (at least one hour) and there have been major problems with both respiratory and cardiac motion which produces artefacts, blurring the image. The development of electro-cardiogram gating techniques to time the scans between cardiac contractions has partially overcome this problem but there is still respiratory motion to eliminate before the technique becomes better than CT for the assessment of lung pathology.

FURTHER READING

Felson B., Wiot J., eds. (1980). *Seminars in Roentgenology*. Vol. 15, 1 & 2.
Felson B., Wiot J., eds. (1988). *Seminars in Roentgenology*. Vol. 23, 1.
Fraser R., Pare P. (1979). *Diagnosis of Diseases of the Chest*. 2nd edn. Philadelphia: W.B. Saunders.

Chapter 5

Ventilatory Dysfunction

AMANDA THOMAS, ELIZABETH ELLIS

INTRODUCTION

Pulmonary ventilation is the result of a series of complex interactions between the central breathing control mechanisms, the muscles responsible for breathing and the skeletal structures they influence. In order to understand these interactions, we have developed a system of analysis (Figure 5.1) that helps the therapist examine ventilation as it occurs under normal and abnormal conditions.

The system presented here has developed out of many attempts to build a consistent framework for analysis and problem-solving in the teaching and implementation of cardiothoracic physiotherapy. This development follows a recent trend in physiotherapy decision-making away from a focus on pathology, towards an analysis based on the functional disorder created by the pathology. This type of analysis is possible since the respiratory system has a number of important functions which include biochemical, immunological and gas exchange functions. The advantage of using this system is that it allows a comprehensive analysis of the effect of changes in respiratory mechanics on the gas exchange function of the lung.

The system is logically sequenced and easily understood and applied. One of the limitations of presenting a system of analysis in this way is that some physiological concepts are oversimplified. For the student starting out in this area, simplifying the analysis is necessary in the initial stages of learning so that more complex analytical skills can be developed.

The System of Analysis

Ventilation is initiated by a neural mechanism termed the *respiratory control centre*. Involuntary respiratory activity is controlled by neural tissue anatomically localized to the medulla and pons of the brainstem.[1] These areas are also connected to the cerebral cortex, providing voluntary control of breathing. The oral regions of the frontal lobe and ventral surface of the temporal lobes have been identified as the cortical locations of voluntary respiratory movements.[2]

Impulses from the respiratory control centre travel along nerves to *respiratory muscles*. Substantial debate exists within the literature as to the precise role of some of the respiratory muscles in producing the commonly observed respiratory movements. For a more detailed explanation of these points the reader is referred to the current literature.[3,4,5,6] However, it has been recognized that the scalenes, diaphragm and intercostal muscles need to be activated together in a coordinated manner for the chest wall and abdomen to move in the way that is described as 'normal'.[4]

Activity of the respiratory muscles determines the movement of the *rib cage* (bone, pleura and lung tissue). Specifically, contraction of the diaphragm causes anteroposterior and transverse displacements of the rib cage. In addition, diaphragmatic descent during inspiration causes a decrease in intra-abdominal volume which increases intra-abdominal pressure, causing the anterior movement of the abdominal wall.[7] Respiratory muscle activity, therefore, also causes changes within the *abdomen*.

The consequences of these movements of the rib cage (thorax) are an increase in thoracic volume and a decrease in intrathoracic pressure. This pressure change causes a net *movement of air* through airways into the lungs. For effective *alveolar ventilation* to occur, the rib cage and abdomen need to be free to move through their normal displacements. Restriction of either the rib cage, abdomen or the movement of air (which may occur as a result of numerous pathologies) results in poor alveolar ventilation and an inability of the respiratory system to maintain normal gas exchange.

Respiratory mechanics must be seen as dynamic rather than static in nature. No one point of analysis, or level within this system can be looked at in isolation, since each level interacts with others. Fortunately, under both

RESPIRATORY CONTROLLER
Involuntary and voluntary control of breathing

activates the

RESPIRATORY MUSCLES
Diaphragm, intercostal and accessory muscles

cause movement of

RIB CAGE　　　　　　　**ABDOMEN**
Bone, pleura, lung tissue　　Pressure changes

resulting in

MOVEMENT OF AIR
Into and out of the lungs

and

ALVEOLAR VENTILATION

Figure 5.1　The interaction of the major components of the system of analysis presented in this chapter.

normal and abnormal circumstances, this dynamic interaction allows the respiratory system to compensate for any extra demands placed on a particular level of the system. For example, during exercise, the total demand for oxygen increases, which requires a higher overall ventilation (both alveolar and dead space ventilation). The system is able to compensate for this greater need for ventilation by increasing neural drive to the respiratory muscles which generate greater intrathoracic pressures and move more air into and out of the lungs. Unfortunately, the ability of the system to compensate eventually reaches a maximum where, despite full compensation by all components of the system, it cannot cope with further increases in the load.

Similarly, when pathology is involved at one level, which increases the stress at that point, other levels of the system compensate to maintain the functions of the lung or to keep alveolar ventilation constant. Often, the system's compensatory strategies are evident as the signs and symptoms of respiratory distress. For example, during an acute asthmatic episode in which the abnormality is in the airways, the body compensates by increasing respiratory muscle effort in an attempt to overcome the increased resistive work of breathing. This is evident by a sensation of breathlessness and increased recruitment of accessory muscles.

Using the Analysis System in Decision-making

Understanding this system of analysis and the complex influence that dysfunction at one point can have on the whole respiratory system provides the basis for physiotherapy decision-making. Physiotherapeutic intervention may need to be directed towards more than one point of the system, as pathology at one level may disturb, or be compensated for at other levels. The skill in planning effective intervention is based on a decision as to which point intervention will be most effective. For example, after abdominal surgery the functional disorder stems from the incision and handling of the abdominal contents. Clinical and experimental evidence supports intervention based on cortical control of breathing, since this intervention is most effective even though it is not aimed directly at the cause of the disorder.

Several factors need to be considered when deciding on the level to which intervention should be directed. Initially, clinical analysis should involve identification of the major focus of disruption to the system and the consequences of this disruption to the other levels of the system. This step should identify the source of the patient's presenting signs and symptoms, since these features appear as a result of compensation for the disturbance.

The next step is to identify which components of disruption to the system are reversible and which are fixed, that is, not amenable to intervention. For example, severe cases of spinal deformity are considered fixed, as there is little that physiotherapy or surgical intervention can do to correct the deformity. Other conditions can be seen as temporarily fixed. For example, severe airways obstruction may take some time to resolve and in the early stages there may be little that physiotherapy can do directly for the underlying problem. The therapist should consider the airways obstruction as temporarily fixed and focus intervention at other points in the system. The notion of reversibility applies to our current knowledge of what factors respond to intervention. The next step is to plan intervention in such a way as to affect not only the major focus of disruption, but other levels as well.

Clinical decisions will be influenced by the nature of the immediate problems identified through the history and examination. At times it is necessary to deal with immediate and uncomfortable situations for the person, e.g., the distress caused by acute dyspnoea. However, as the person's comfort and signs and symptoms improve, other strategies can be selected that will either deal directly or indirectly with the underlying cause of the individual's complaint.

The following sections will serve to illustrate the application of this system of analysis to clinical practice. The interactions occurring throughout the system due to a dysfunction at a particular level of the system are described in detail, and the planning and implementation of physiotherapeutic intervention discussed. It should be noted here that the following text describes examples of the application of this system of analysis, and is not meant to be an exhaustive reference to all possible circumstances. There will be other factors identified through history-taking and physical examination that will need to be considered in the clinical environment.

RESPIRATORY CONTROLLER

The respiratory centres of the mid-brain may be affected by a number of mechanisms, such as tumours, infections, cerebrovascular accidents or by congenital abnormalities such as primary alveolar hypoventilation. In addition, cortical control of ventilation may be affected by similar abnormalities. For example, voluntary control over breathing may be difficult in the presence of some cortical lesions. Abnormalities in respiratory control can cause a variety of disturbances throughout the respiratory system which can ultimately cause alveolar hypoventilation. Analysis of the presenting signs and symptoms may give some clue as to the location and nature of the lesion. For example, pontine lesions may be indicated by an apneustic pattern of breathing which means that the patient pauses at the end of inspiration, and in some patients expiratory pauses may also be present.

Assessment features may vary considerably and because isolated lesions of the brain stem are relatively uncommon they are often difficult to diagnose. None the less the common clinical signs are eventually those of chronic hypoventilation and the control of breathing is often worse during sleep, particularly rapid eye movement sleep. Symptoms may relate to sleep disturbances such as daytime sleepiness and fatigue. Morning headaches, transient loss of consciousness and abnormal ventilatory response to exertion may all occur as a result of ineffective automatic mechanisms controlling breathing.

Management is aimed at providing an appropriate level of ventilatory support. Problems of control of breathing as a cause of respiratory failure are identified with detailed studies of ventilatory control and breathing during sleep. These studies help define the nature and extent of the underlying problem.

RESPIRATORY MUSCLES

Respiratory muscle function can be affected by diseases which act directly on the muscle or indirectly via the motor pathways of the central and peripheral nervous systems. Conditions which affect the muscles directly include such categories as the muscular dystrophies, especially the limb girdle and Duchenne types, and myopathies such as glycogen storage diseases, polymyositis and myotonia dystrophy. Conditions which affect the motor pathways include spinal cord injury, poliomyelitis and a range of neuropathies.

A case description of an individual with acute idiopathic polyneuritis or Guillain–Barré syndrome, which is a neuropathy of unknown cause, is considered in detail below.

Characteristics of Guillain–Barré

A person with Guillain–Barré syndrome will present with a history of rapidly progressing muscle weakness which may have a pattern of ascending progression; that is, the weakness may start in the lower limbs and work upwards. In the advanced stages, the respiratory muscles become involved. This leads to reduced chest wall expansion bilaterally and reduced air entry. Fine crackles may be heard at the end of inspiration. There may be other signs of progressive respiratory failure as the weakness progresses, such as cyanosis, or headaches due to carbon dioxide retention. There may be no other respiratory abnormality, particularly if the person is young and has no history of smoking or chronic lung disease.

Lung function testing will typically show reduced lung volumes in a restricted pattern. When vital capacity (VC) falls below 1.0 litre, assisted ventilation is considered. Reduced respiratory muscle strength will be evident on measurement of maximal inspiratory and expiratory pressures at the mouth. In addition, loss of lung volume particularly in the bases of the lungs will be seen on radiography. Arterial blood gas analysis may show worsening hypoxaemia and hypercapnia as the condition progresses.

Analysis. In this condition, there is progressive muscle weakness involving the respiratory muscles leading to reduced thoracic movement and reduced airflow (Figure 5.2). Signs of alveolar hypoventilation appear as the weakness progresses and this may lead to respiratory failure.

At the level of muscle function it is known that the underlying pathology affecting the muscles is only reversible with time, as specific medical treatment is not, as yet, available. Thus, the underlying condition is considered temporarily irreversible to intervention and physiotherapy must focus on the consequences of this problem for the rest of the system.

Treatment Planning. Intervention should be planned with the rate of progress of the disorder taken into consideration. Careful reassessment prior to each treatment is necessary to assess this rate of progress. The goal of treatment would be to provide sufficient ventilatory support to allow adequate gas exchange and to prevent complications developing such as atelectasis. If the person has previously been in good health, all effort should be made to preserve lung function and prevent damage occurring secondary to the muscle involvement.

If ventilatory support is instituted as a part of overall management, then one goal of treatment would be to maximize the distribution of the assisted ventilation by ensuring adequate positional changes and careful monitoring of the individual's response to ventilation, through frequent assessment of

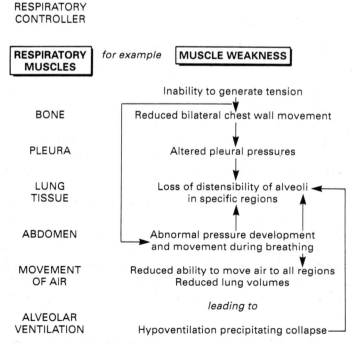

Figure 5.2 The consequences of Guillain–Barré, an example of muscle weakness, on the major components of the respiratory system.

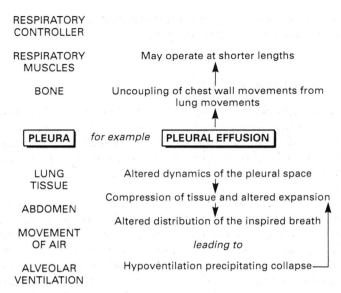

RESPIRATORY
CONTROLLER

RESPIRATORY   May operate at shorter lengths
   MUSCLES   ↑

     BONE   Uncoupling of chest wall movements from
                            lung movements
                                 ↑

   PLEURA   *for example*   PLEURAL EFFUSION

     LUNG   Altered dynamics of the pleural space
    TISSUE   ↓
                  Compression of tissue and altered expansion
  ABDOMEN   ↓
                  Altered distribution of the inspired breath
 MOVEMENT
   OF AIR   *leading to*

  ALVEOLAR   Hypoventilation precipitating collapse
 VENTILATION

Figure 5.3   The consequences of a pleural effusion, an example of dysfunction of the pleural component of the thorax, on the major components of the respiratory system.

air entry, arterial blood gases and chest radiograph. Other goals include preventing the complications of intubation such as tracheal irritation and altered mucociliary clearance, and preventing the problems associated with prolonged immobility, such as muscle shortening.

THE THORAX AND ABDOMEN

As previously noted, respiratory muscle activity causes movement and pressure changes in the thorax and abdomen. The thorax has been divided into three components, the bony structures, the pleura and the lung tissue itself. Each of these components, and the abdomen, has the potential to disrupt the respiratory system's maintenance of normal alveolar ventilation. In this section, the consequences of abnormal mechanics of the thorax or abdomen are illustrated. For example, the *pleural component* of the thorax can be the cause of respiratory dysfunction when normal pleural mechanics are disrupted. The pleural tissue can become stiff or fibrosed with certain diseases, or the pleural space can become filled with air as in pneumothorax. Figure 5.3 illustrates the consequences of disruption to pleural mechanics when the pleural space is occupied by fluid, as in a pleural effusion.

The *bony components* of the thorax, i.e., the skeletal rib cage and rib articulations, can influence respiratory function when they are directly affected by trauma, disease or congenital deformity. An example of a slowly progressive deformity of the spine and skeletal rib cage, known as kyphoscoliosis, will be used to illustrate this point.

Characteristics of Kyphoscoliosis

As a result of the spinal and rib cage deformity there is usually reduced chest wall movement with increased abdominal wall movement. As a result of the severely distorted chest wall, air entry is reduced asymmetrically. The person may complain of reduced exercise tolerance usually limited by dyspnoea. This can become progressively more debilitating with the severity of the deformity.

Lung function testing will show reduced lung volumes in a restrictive pattern, with very little effect on expiratory flow rates. Chest wall compliance will be reduced, although there may not be any primary lung stiffness. Respiratory muscle strength measurements may show decreased inspiratory pressures and near normal expiratory pressures. Blood gas analysis initially may show mild hypoxaemia and moderate hypercapnia. This may progress with time. There may be slight hyperinflation of areas of one lung and loss of volume in the other and the spinal and rib cage deformity will be seen on radiography.

Analysis. The primary level of dysfunction in this case, is the abnormality of the bony components of the rib cage (Figure 5.4). Spinal curvature can cause a gross distortion of the rib cage. This leads to a reduced range of movement

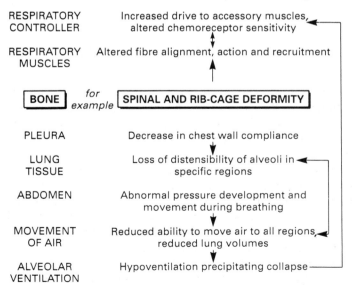

Figure 5.4 The consequences of kyphoscoliosis, an example of dysfunction of the bone component of the thorax, on the major components of the respiratory system.

of the costovertebral joints and respiratory movement of the ribs is reduced. Chest wall compliance therefore decreases. Secondary to the rib-cage deformity, the diaphragm no longer inserts with its normal fibre alignment along the costal margin. Hence, reduced inspiratory pressures are generated and accessory muscles are recruited to compensate for the ineffective diaphragm. Alveolar hypoventilation eventually occurs which predisposes the person to the respiratory complications of collapse and infection and causes a ventilation/perfusion mismatch.

During the early stages of kyphoscoliosis, respiratory control centres may not be affected, although there appears to be an increased drive to the accessory muscles which is probably associated with the mild respiratory failure evident on blood gas analysis. While daytime resting symptoms may not be clinically severe, the inability of the respiratory system to cope with increasing activity levels or different sleep states can reveal more severe alveolar hypoventilation. For example, during rapid eye movement (REM) sleep, there is an inhibition of the accessory muscles of breathing. The work of breathing falls largely to the diaphragm, which is dysfunctional. This causes even less movement of the rib cage and abdominal wall. The person, therefore, moves little or no air into the lungs during REM sleep. This is a form of sleep apnoea. Acute alveolar hypoventilation occurs which eventually rouses the person from REM sleep. Sleep fragmentation occurs over a long period of time and the individual eventually accommodates to higher and higher levels of carbon dioxide (CO_2) until CO_2 retention occurs during the awake state as well. This chronic resetting of the chemoreceptors may contribute significantly to the hypoventilation seen in end stage chest wall deformities.[8]

Treatment planning. The analysis of this situation is again dependent on the reversibility or otherwise of each component. The spinal deformity is the key disturbance of the system and is reversible surgically when identified early and before severe respiratory complications set in. Usually by the time the person is in chronic respiratory failure surgery is not possible and the deformity is considered irreversible. Braces and jackets have been used to stabilize the deterioration with varied success.[9] The integrity of the chest wall should be preserved as much as possible with regular exercise, with the goal of maintaining the mobility of the rib cage and vertebrae. If the spinal deformity is irreversible, the respiratory muscle alignment is unlikely to be altered with any specific intervention. Diaphragm function may be improved in terms of strength and endurance with specific respiratory exercises (see Chapter 7). However, this has not been demonstrated conclusively in this group of people.

The complications of REM hypoventilation can be prevented with assisted ventilation during sleep using non-invasive ventilatory support. Assisted ventilation at night will reverse the desensitization of the control centres and improve the daytime awake alveolar ventilation.[10]

The *lung tissue* component of the thorax can be directly affected by a number of diseases, infective and inflammatory states. These problems directly interfere with the ability of the lung to achieve normal gas exchange and cause the system to respond by adopting compensatory strategies. These strategies are illustrated by examining the effect of lung tissue inflammation on respiratory function such as occurs in pneumonia and the effect of stiffening of the lung tissue as in tissue fibrosis (Figure 5.5).

Characteristics of Pneumonia

The individual with pneumonia invariably has a cough. This cough can be dry and irritating or productive of a wide spectrum of sputum type and colour, depending on the site, type and stage of disease. For example, lobar or segmental pneumonia is characterized by bloodstained, rusty sputum. An associated pleuritic type chest pain, worse with coughing and deep inspiration is often reported. The person may also report fever, shivering, general malaise, nausea, vomiting and a decrease in exercise tolerance due to shortness of breath.

Physical examination can reveal cyanosis, an increase in respiratory rate and a pattern of breathing confined to the upper chest. Some accessory muscle recruitment may be noted. Auscultation reveals a decrease in air entry or bronchial breath sounds over localized parts of the chest wall. The percussion note will also be dull over these areas. In many cases there is a degree of hypoxaemia and an elevated temperature.

After two to four days of inflammation a consolidated area is usually

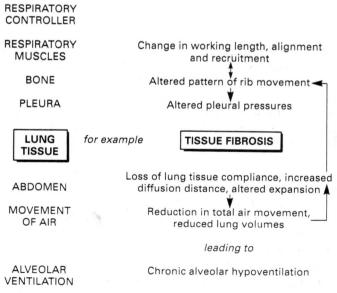

Figure 5.5   *The consequences of pulmonary fibrosis, an example of dysfunction of the lung tissue component of the thorax, on the major components of the respiratory system.*

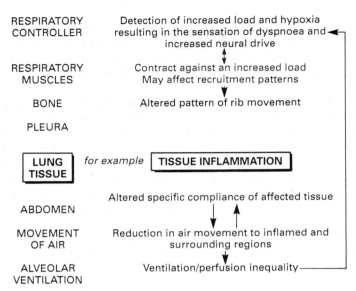

RESPIRATORY
CONTROLLER
Detection of increased load and hypoxia
resulting in the sensation of dyspnoea and
increased neural drive

RESPIRATORY
MUSCLES
Contract against an increased load
May affect recruitment patterns

BONE
Altered pattern of rib movement

PLEURA

LUNG
TISSUE
for example
TISSUE INFLAMMATION

Altered specific compliance of affected tissue
ABDOMEN

MOVEMENT
OF AIR
Reduction in air movement to inflamed and
surrounding regions

ALVEOLAR
VENTILATION
Ventilation/perfusion inequality

Figure 5.6 The consequences of pneumonia, an example of lung tissue inflammation, on the major components of the respiratory system.

evident on the chest radiograph and the appearance of this consolidation changes as the pneumonia progresses through its various stages.

Analysis. Pneumonia refers to the process of inflammation of the alveoli. There are a variety of types and causes of pneumonia and the reader is referred to a general medical textbook for a full description of these factors. For this discussion, it is assumed that the effects of alveoli inflammation are generally the same regardless of the cause and type of organism involved (Figure 5.6).

Inflammatory responses are always associated with the production of exudate due to vasodilatation and an increased permeability of blood vessels in the region. In the lung, exudate collects within the alveoli replacing space which is normally reserved for air. When many alveoli become filled with fluid the specific lung region involved becomes increasingly difficult to expand since its compliance is altered. This change in compliance of the region also alters the distensibility of the surrounding lung tissue. These changes cause alveolar hypoventilation of the pneumonic region and its surrounds which helps to explain the existence of the radiological and auscultatory findings. In addition, the inflammatory reactions of the lung tissue can cause an inflammatory response in the surrounding pleura which explains the pleuritic chest pain.

Alteration in the specific compliance of the affected region causes the respiratory muscles to contract harder to generate the same pressures, since they must pull against greater resistive and elastic loads. This may cause the neural perception of an abnormal inspiratory load and trigger the sensation of dyspnoea. Finally, a large area of non-ventilated lung tissue may cause a ventilation/perfusion mismatch and result in arterial hypoxaemia. Hypoxia may trigger respiratory centre reflexes, which may alter the person's pattern of breathing as a response to the increased neural drive.

Treatment planning. Identification of the stage of the inflammatory process in pneumonia is essential to justify physiotherapy intervention in individuals with this problem. The primary treatment for pneumonia is the administration of pharmacotherapeutic agents specific to the virus, bacteria or organism causing the inflammation. Therefore, in the early stages of the process, the problem at the alveoli level is temporarily irreversible by physiotherapy intervention. Pharmacological agents are required to assist the body's natural defence mechanisms to break down the consolidated region.

Treatment at this point would be aimed at reversing loss of volume in adjacent lung segments, preventing further collapse, and preventing gross ventilation/perfusion mismatching by using various body positions to increase the volume of the affected parts of lung (see Appendix B) and alter the distribution of ventilation. The aggressiveness of techniques chosen for these reversible components will depend on the severity of the presenting symptoms, in particular the presence of pain. There is evidence which suggests that the use of positive end-expiratory pressure (PEEP) and continuous positive airways pressure (CPAP) can be effective in aiding the re-expansion of atelectatic lung and preventing further airways collapse.[11]

Once the pneumonia has progressed into its resolution and healing phase, the problem at the alveoli level can be viewed as reversible, since it should now be possible to assist the removal of debris from the affected alveoli and re-ventilate collapsed lung units. It has not, however, been demonstrated that traditional physiotherapeutic techniques of secretion removal are effective in hastening the resolution of the pneumonia.[12,13] Once the consolidation has begun to resolve, techniques to assist the removal of secretions may, however, be of value to the individual.

It should be noted that while pneumonia can be seen in otherwise normal individuals, it is more commonly observed in people with a lowered resistance to infection. These include the aged, those recovering from surgery or blunt trauma to the chest, young children, and those with pre-existing lung disease. The process of physiotherapy decision-making in these cases will need to be based on a careful analysis of the combined consequences of two or more disturbances at different levels of the system.

Changes to the *abdominal compartment* itself can disturb the mechanical interaction that exists between the thorax and abdomen. The compliance of the abdomen can be altered when its volume is increased by air, peritoneal fluid (Figure 5.7), faeces, blood or pregnancy. Direct trauma to the abdomen in the form of surgery also disrupts its normal interaction with the thorax. This issue is examined through illustration of the respiratory consequences of upper abdominal surgery.

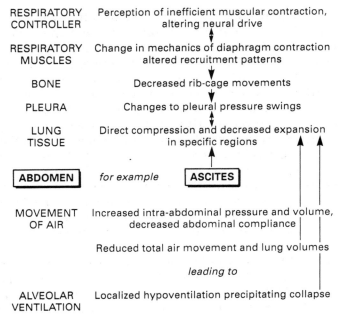

RESPIRATORY   Perception of inefficient muscular contraction,
CONTROLLER   altering neural drive

RESPIRATORY   Change in mechanics of diaphragm contraction
MUSCLES   altered recruitment patterns

BONE   Decreased rib-cage movements

PLEURA   Changes to pleural pressure swings

LUNG   Direct compression and decreased expansion
TISSUE   in specific regions

ABDOMEN   *for example*   ASCITES

MOVEMENT   Increased intra-abdominal pressure and volume,
OF AIR   decreased abdominal compliance

Reduced total air movement and lung volumes

leading to

ALVEOLAR   Localized hypoventilation precipitating collapse
VENTILATION

Figure 5.7   The consequences of ascites, an example of dysfunction at the level of the abdomen, on the major components of the respiratory system.

Characteristics of Respiratory Dysfunction after Upper Abdominal Surgery

Following upper abdominal surgery, it is common to observe an alteration to the normal pattern of breathing, which may include a reduction in anterior abdominal wall displacement and lateral chest wall movement, as well as an increase in upper rib cage movement. These changes are observed during both quiet and deep breathing. Breath sounds may be reduced in basal lung regions, as will the percussion note heard over these regions.

Clinical investigations in individuals following upper abdominal surgery consistently demonstrate a reduction in both static (VC and FRC) and dynamic (FVC and FEV_1) lung function tests. Chest radiographs may reveal some degree of diaphragm elevation and loss of volume in the basal lung regions.

Analysis. Surgery via an incision through the anterior abdominal wall causes the variety of abnormalities outlined above. These abnormalities can be attributed to:

1   the effects of anaesthesia on respiratory function;
2   the effects of the incision, and
3   poor or absent diaphragm function (Figure 5.8).

The nature of diaphragm dysfunction after upper abdominal surgery has been the topic of numerous investigations; however, the precise cause has yet to be elucidated. The inspiratory action of the diaphragm on the abdomen is to cause a forward displacement of the anterior abdominal wall, brought about by the increase in abdominal pressure resulting from diaphragm descent.[14] Following upper abdominal surgery, investigators have demonstrated a reduction in the inspiratory movement of the anterior abdominal wall in both humans and dogs.[15,16,17] The reduced movement correlates with a decrease in abdominal pressure swings during inspiration.[17] In some subjects, abdominal pressure swings occur in the opposite direction to that normally observed, that is, the abdominal or gastric pressure becomes negative instead of positive.

The observed changes in anterior abdominal wall movement and abdominal pressure probably reflect decreased movement of the diaphragm. In fact the parameters used directly to measure diaphragm function, or the diaphragm's contribution to inspiration, invariably show decreased values after upper abdominal surgery. These measures include the transdiaphragmatic pressure (Pdi), the maximal transdiaphragmatic pressure (Pdi_{max}) and the ratio of pressure in the abdomen (Pab) to the transdiaphragmatic pressure (Pab/Pdi).[15,16,17,18] Reports of the length of time these pressure changes persist vary within the literature. Some reports consider a return to normal values occurs after 24 hours,[17] while others suggest that control values are not reached until seven days after the operation.[16]

Reduced diaphragm activity during inspiration is also reflected in the decreased static and dynamic lung volumes recorded. Of particular interest

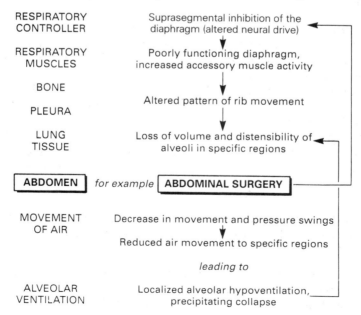

Figure 5.8 The consequences of upper abdominal surgery on the major components of the respiratory system.

is the dramatic reduction in the vital capacity and total lung capacity. This decrease in lung volume, combined with the upper chest pattern of breathing, may alter the distribution of the inspired breath toward non-dependent regions.[19] This may help to explain the existence of the basal alveolar hypoventilation and atelectasis found clinically.

It has been considered that postoperative pain associated with the abdominal incision and surgical process may be the cause of the diaphragm dysfunction observed in this group of people. However, several investigations have demonstrated that even when pain is adequately controlled by epidural anaesthesia,[16,20] reduction in diaphragm function persists.

Recent work into the nature of the diaphragm dysfunction after upper abdominal surgery suggests that a reflex arising from the abdominal viscera may cause diaphragmatic inhibition during quiet breathing and maximal voluntary efforts.[21] Since diaphragm contractility itself appears to be preserved in these individuals,[18] it is suggested that the reflex inhibition may be mediated by supraspinal centres, decreasing the output to the diaphragm during breathing. The exact nature of this neural reflex remains to be fully explained.

Treatment planning. The predominant problem arising from the mechanical abnormalities described above is alveolar hypoventilation, particularly of the more dependent lung regions or those closest to the poorly functioning diaphragm in the upright posture. In people who have pre-existing respiratory risk factors, the inability to develop sufficient expiratory pressures in order to produce an effective cough may also predispose them to the problems associated with secretion retention. For the purposes of this discussion an assumption will be made that alveolar hypoventilation is the primary dysfunction and this will therefore be our main focus.

The physiotherapist needs to determine which aspects of the underlying cause of the alveolar hypoventilation are reversible and which are non-reversible. This process requires a decision regarding the reversibility of the abnormal postoperative respiratory function, including diaphragmatic inhibition, if present. This decision, in turn will influence the short- and long-term goals of management.

In situations where there are few indicators of voluntary diaphragmatic activity (lack of lateral chest wall and abdominal movement during voluntary attempts to increase lung volume), the therapist may assume that diaphragmatic inhibition is occurring. Attempts to improve alveolar hypoventilation that are independent of diaphragm activity may need to be selected in some cases where voluntary efforts are ineffective. Passive means of inflation (intermittent positive-pressure breathing) and of altering the distribution of ventilation by positioning are methods used clinically to reduce alveolar hypoventilation in these people. The implementation of these techniques implies a passive role for the patient. However, in the presence of a dysfunctional diaphragm, these techniques may be the only methods of reducing the complications of hypoventilation.

If diaphragm dysfunction is the cause of the predominant problem in these patients, intervention should be aimed ideally at improving the function of the diaphragm. The goal of treatment would be to improve alveolar hypoventilation by improving control of the diaphragm, rather than simply increasing lung volume. Such an intervention will involve techniques designed to overcome the inhibition of the diaphragm by higher centres, since overcoming the inhibition should restore diaphragmatic function. These techniques are based on the same principles advocated for the practice of everyday activities in people with poor motor control. Treatment may entail encouraging the person to overcome the inhibition by selective voluntary attempts to achieve a diaphragmatic contraction. The therapist's hand position, verbal instruction, encouragement, feedback and frequent practice may be the important determinants of the effectiveness of this intervention. The ability of a person to override a central inhibition of the diaphragm by consciously attending to the action has not been systematically evaluated.

The therapist may choose to employ a combination of the above approaches in the treatment of respiratory dysfunction after upper abdominal surgery. Passive techniques may be necessary initially to reinforce the goal of the desired movements, and to encourage the person actively to participate in the act of increasing lung volume. Some form of evaluation of voluntary diaphragmatic activity must be employed to determine the time of return of normal function. The literature suggests that seven days after surgery the inhibition may still exist.[16] The decision as to which level of intervention is selected must therefore influence not only the techniques employed, but also the manner in which they are utilized.

MOVEMENT OF AIR THROUGH AIRWAYS

Air movement within the airways is dependent on the nature of intrapulmonary pressure changes brought about by respiratory muscle action and movement of the thorax and abdomen. Airflow can be disturbed within the airways when changes take place that prevent air moving at normal velocities or prevent it from moving at all, for example, when the airway is blocked by a foreign body such as an inhaled peanut. Airways may become narrowed such as in asthma, where bronchoconstriction narrows the tubes through which the air passes. Excessive amounts of pulmonary secretions within the airways have a similar effect on altering airflow velocity since they produce a generalized or local obstruction to the movement of air. The effect of a disturbance of air movement on the rest of the respiratory system is illustrated by examining examples of this problem, first as an acute episode (asthma) and secondly as a slowly progressive chronic disease of the airways (chronic airflow limitation).

Characteristics of Acute Asthma

The person with severe acute asthma will appear to be in some distress and complain of dyspnoea, initially on exertion, later progressing to breathlessness at rest. The person will demonstrate marked recruitment of accessory muscles of breathing. Despite this increase in respiratory effort, there will be reduced overall chest wall movement and a change in the normal pattern of breathing. The thorax may be hyperinflated and the percussion note will be hyper-resonant. The volume of air in the lungs tends to be relatively static as very little air entry may be heard. On the other hand, expiratory wheezes will be heard, even in mild cases and inspiratory wheezing will become evident as the condition progresses. An audible wheeze at the mouth and a dry harsh cough are also common.

Lung function tests demonstrate an obstructive pattern with a markedly reduced FEV_1 relative to the FVC, peak expiratory flow rates (PEFR), and the flow recorded after 50% of the VC ($\dot{V}_{50}$). Arterial blood gas analysis will show a mild hypoxaemia and initially, normal carbon dioxide levels which may progress to hypercapnia as the condition worsens. Chest radiographs may show progressive degrees of hyperinflation. However, in uncomplicated cases there may be very little else evident radiographically.

Analysis. The pathology of asthma, that is, smooth muscle spasm, mucosal inflammation and increased secretion production, causes the airways to narrow and this causes both increased resistance to airflow and early airways closure. The early airways closure occurs because higher intra-thoracic pressures are required to achieve expiratory flow through narrow airways. These higher pressures result in greater collapsing pressures acting on the airways. In addition, as the internal diameter of the airway is reduced, they are more likely to close during expiration with a given collapsing pressure. There is, therefore, an increased closing volume.

This early closing pattern may lead to both passive and active processes occurring (Figure 5.9). Early closure pattern leads to 'passive' gas trapping and an increase in the alveolar volume at the end of expiration. During each inspiration, as the airways open, alveoli fill with air. As the airways close on expiration that air becomes trapped. This process continues, increasing the size of the alveoli until the pressure in the alveoli is such that it can resist the collapsing forces and allow some flow of air in and out. This process results in hyperinflation or an increase in the FRC which is the volume of air left in the lung at the end of a tidal breath. The consequence of hyperinflation is that the chest wall and abdominal shape are changed and the respiratory muscles must operate at altered lengths. Most importantly, the inspiratory muscles are working from a shortened length. The muscles do not act as efficiently at the shortened length and this can lead to an increased recruitment of inspiratory accessory muscles.

The 'active' mechanism which occurs as a consequence of gas trapping is mediated by arterial blood gas abnormalities secondary to ineffective gas

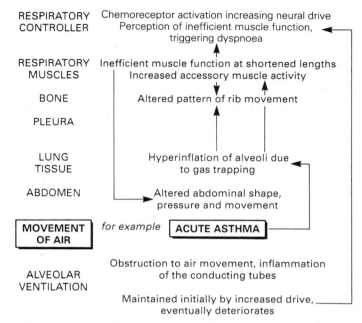

RESPIRATORY   Chemoreceptor activation increasing neural drive
CONTROLLER   Perception of inefficient muscle function,
                                    triggering dyspnoea

RESPIRATORY   Inefficient muscle function at shortened lengths
MUSCLES   Increased accessory muscle activity

BONE   Altered pattern of rib movement

PLEURA

LUNG   Hyperinflation of alveoli due
TISSUE   to gas trapping

ABDOMEN   Altered abdominal shape,
                                    pressure and movement

MOVEMENT   *for example*   ACUTE ASTHMA
OF AIR

                        Obstruction to air movement, inflammation
ALVEOLAR   of the conducting tubes
VENTILATION
                        Maintained initially by increased drive,
                               eventually deteriorates

Figure 5.9   The consequences of acute increases in airways resistance, or asthma, an example of dysfunction at the level of air movement, on the major components of the respiratory system.

exchange. Hypoxaemia and hypercapnia are detected by the central and peripheral chemoreceptors which respond by increasing drive to the respiratory muscles. Increased inspiratory muscle drive will result in recruitment of the accessory muscles and allow the maintenance of a high FRC. In addition, the hypoxic response of the carotid bodies will trigger an alarm or arousal response which contributes to the distress and perception of dyspnoea.

Adequate gas exchange may be maintained by an increase in respiratory muscle effort, particularly if the airway resistance is mild. As obstruction to airflow becomes greater and the FRC increases, the work of breathing increases. Eventually, the oxygen cost of maintaining ventilation may become greater than any increase in oxygen uptake afforded by the level of ventilation and it becomes inefficient to try and maintain that level of ventilation. At this time, the level of arterial carbon dioxide starts to rise and the person is in danger of deteriorating rapidly.

Treatment planning. The critical bronchoconstriction component of acute asthma is usually reversible with drug therapy, and when this occurs all the other levels of dysfunction will reverse accordingly. Therefore, the most important level to affect is that of air movement through the airways. The overall aim is to improve the movement of air which can most efficiently be achieved by the administration of drug therapy, such as bronchodilators and corticosteroids. The initial aims of physiotherapy intervention are:

1 To assist in the administration of inhaled drug therapy, by ensuring that an even distribution of the drug occurs throughout the lungs by varying the pattern of breathing;
2 To assist the person cope with the symptoms of asthma such as dyspnoea, while drug therapy is taking effect.

The physiotherapist can provide the person with strategies to reduce the dyspnoea such as supported positioning and relaxation methods. Until some improvement has been achieved at the level of the airways, there is no evidence that altering the pattern of breathing or the compensatory recruitment of the respiratory muscles has any benefit.

While secretions are not necessarily a feature of early acute asthma, careful reassessment with time will reveal whether to include techniques to facilitate removal of secretions. These may be particularly relevant if the episode of asthma has been associated with a lower respiratory tract infection.

A long-term goal of intervention is the prevention of further episodes of asthma. Education on healthy lifestyle, self management and reducing exposure to allergens can be included in a comprehensive programme of asthma management.

Characteristics of Chronic Airflow Limitation

The clinical picture of chronic airflow limitation (CAL) is the result of a variety of pathological changes associated with the underlying disease processes. It is important to recognize that the presenting signs and symptoms of CAL are at times due to an acute exacerbation of an underlying chronic problem. The following descriptions represent combinations of signs and symptoms that may be observed to varying degrees in the chronic condition with or without an acute infection. Not all persons with CAL will present with all the abnormalities described.

The person with CAL invariably reports a limitation or decline in exercise capacity. This decline is usually due to shortness of breath or dyspnoea that is brought on by minimal exertion. In severe cases, dyspnoea may be present at rest. It is not uncommon for dyspnoea to have a cardiac origin as well as a pulmonary origin.

On physical examination the person may display changes in chest wall shape and movement. The chest may be chronically altered into a 'barrel' shape, that is, with an increase in the anteroposterior chest diameter. The movement of the lateral chest wall may be reduced or paradoxical,[22] while the movement of the upper chest will predominate in the breathing pattern. Depending on the extent and nature of the underlying disease, there may be abnormalities of abdominal wall movement. In some cases it may be absent or even paradoxical, that is, moving inward instead of outward during inspiration. Inspection of the nail beds and skin may reveal peripheral cyanosis, or central cyanosis may be seen in the mucous membranes, particularly the mouth and tongue. The skin may appear pale, papery or dry and an abnormal curvature of the nails known as 'clubbing' may occur. Auscultation may reveal various combinations of lung sounds. Reduced or turbulent breath sounds may be heard over the entire chest wall combined with widespread expiratory wheezes, particularly during expiration. Hyperresonance may be noted on percussion.

Clinical investigations in this group of people can reflect significant increases in static lung volumes, particularly the residual volume. Dynamic lung volumes are reduced and the flow-volume curve recorded from these people has a typical 'scooped out' appearance (page 37). The chest radiograph may demonstrate hyperinflation. The lung fields may appear translucent, with a loss of visible lung markings.

Analysis. A review of the information presented above indicates that CAL is a complex disorder in which many levels of the analysis system we have presented are dysfunctional. Air movement has been chosen as the level from which to commence this discussion as it appears to be the level of the initial pathological changes (Figure 5.10).

The initial pathological disturbances to the airways and lung tissue in people with CAL are similar to those changes in asthma; however it appears that the actual cause of obstruction differs between people and may represent a combination of pathological changes.[23] These changes include inflammatory processes of the airways in which the bronchial walls are swollen, the bronchial smooth muscle is contracted, and bronchial glands

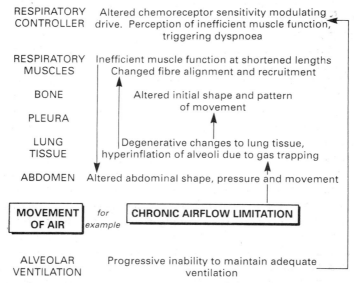

Figure 5.10   *The cascade of abnormalities affecting the major components of the respiratory system due to a dysfunction at the level of air movement known as chronic airflow limitation.*

hypertrophy. In addition to these, degenerative changes occur within the lung parenchyma as a response to chronic inflammation. Chronic loss of lung tissue and destruction of the alveoli wall cause a decrease in the lungs' ability to recoil after inflation.

These two factors (resistance to expiratory airflow and loss of elastic recoil) result in less gas escaping from the lungs before a new inspiration is commenced. As with the acute airways obstruction of asthma, gas becomes trapped in alveoli causing them to hyperinflate.

Since chronic hyperinflation permanently prevents the diaphragm and other respiratory muscles from adopting their normal resting length, adaptive shortening is likely to occur. This has been demonstrated in hamster diaphragm,[24] and is likely to occur in humans as well.[25] It is not the purpose of this discussion to deal in detail with abnormal diaphragmatic function in hyperinflation, as it is covered adequately elsewhere.[6,26,27] However, attempts to contract the diaphragm at high lung volumes is largely responsible for the movement abnormalities demonstrated in the chest wall and abdomen in these people.[28] When the diaphragm contracts at a shortened fibre length its ability to increase intra-abdominal pressure is poor. The accessory and intercostal muscles compensate by assuming much of the work of breathing in these situations.[29] Since their contraction causes large negative pleural pressures, the diaphragm may be 'sucked up' during inspiration. This increases intra-abdominal volume and decreases its pressure. The fall in intra-abdominal pressure is reflected by inward (or paradoxical) movement of the abdomen during the inspiratory cycle.[27]

The mechanical dysfunction described has adverse consequences on the system's ability to maintain adequate ventilation. In addition to this, loss of lung tissue causes a ventilation/perfusion inequality. The compensatory increased work of breathing of the accessory and intercostal muscles may accentuate the demand for available oxygen supply in the face of an inability sufficiently to increase supply. It seems that people with CAL will eventually develop chronic alveolar hypoventilation. This occurs when the system's ability to compensate for the chronic disturbance is exhausted. Some people will then experience adaptive changes in central chemoreceptor sensitivity and tolerance to hypoxaemia and hypercapnia, which appears to be worsened by alcohol consumption.[30]

With adaptation, the system becomes less sensitive to subtle changes in arterial blood gases. This relative insensitivity may actually reduce the drive to the respiratory muscles. Analysis of the model presented demonstrates the effect this has on potentiating the mechanical dysfunction affecting alveolar ventilation, since a decreased respiratory drive to already poorly functioning muscles is potentially dangerous.

Treatment planning. Goals of management will be determined by the particular compensatory strategies which are thought to be responsible for producing the symptoms at the time of treatment. The above analysis suggests that airflow obstruction is the underlying disturbance responsible for the cascade of compensations and the resulting abnormalities outlined. We will limit this discussion to factors that may need to be considered in the decision-making process.

The reversible components of airflow obstruction may be seen as:

1 Decreasing the inflammatory response of the airways.
2 Removing secretions (if present) which may be causing an obstruction to airflow.

The first factor involves administration of bronchodilators and anti-inflammatory agents via inhalation therapy. These will only be effective if the person is able to tolerate and can perform inhalation techniques appropriately. A goal of physiotherapy management may be to ensure the person is familiar with and is effective in their form of manual drug administration.

The second factor, the volume of secretions, is likely to vary considerably. However, even small amounts of secretions may cause significant problems for a person who is very hyperinflated, since coughing may be ineffective. The inability to remove secretions can further cause an obstruction to airflow. The reader is referred to Chapter 6 which deals with secretion removal techniques.

The irreversible component has already been identified as the loss of airway integrity or loss of elastic recoil. Therapy may be directed at assisting the person to cope with the consequences of this problem, e.g., dyspnoea. Various body positions have been found to reduce the subjective feeling of dyspnoea in selected groups of people with CAL. These include high side lying, forward lean in standing and sitting, and supine.[31,32,33] Recent evidence has demonstrated a relationship between these positions, an improved function of the diaphragm, and a reduced activity of the cervical accessory muscles.[33]

Multidisciplinary rehabilitation programmes are suggested as centres of referral for this group of people.[34] These programmes may provide a variety of services including psychological counselling, work modification, general body and specific respiratory muscle training. The latter two aspects are directed toward improving exercise tolerance and the person's perception of dyspnoea and have been shown to have varying degrees of success.[35–40] The reader is referred to Chapter 7 for a detailed discussion of this issue.

CONCLUSION

The system of analysis presented in this chapter is one which we have found useful in understanding the influence of pathology on the components of the respiratory system and how they interrelate. The analysis system enables the therapist to interpret the signs and symptoms of an individual's illness in terms of the initial disturbance and the cascade of effects on other components of the respiratory system. In addition, the system of analysis clarifies the process by which appropriate intervention is selected and provides a rationale for the intervention.

In this chapter, problems have been discussed as if they exist in isolation. In many clinical situations, however, patients will present with a combination of problems, e.g., pneumonia, pleural effusion and postoperative respiratory dysfunction, or altered respiratory function following stroke in a person with CAL. In these cases, the analysis involved will be more complex and require an understanding of each particular dysfunction and how each, in combination, causes the abnormalities observed. Using this analysis will enable the therapist to select an intervention which takes into account the reversibility or otherwise of the combined problems.

It should also be noted that, although the discussion has focused on intervention at the level which has the greatest probability of improving the underlying problem, intervention could be focused upon several levels at the same time. In addition, an intervention may be selected because it has the potential to affect more than one level. Alternatively, a combination of interventions may need to be selected in order comprehensively to manage a dysfunction at one level. If, for example, the therapist is referred a patient with acute CAL, it may be necessary to direct intervention toward different pathological mechanisms at the level of air movement. The therapist may assist in the removal of excessive secretions which may be obstructing the lumen and also ensure effective drug therapy through optimal bronchodilator technique. The skill in decision-making rests with an understanding of the effects of the specific interventions in question and their measured ability to deal with the underlying problem.

As in other areas of physiotherapy practice, it is important to reassess over time the changes which may occur as the result of either progress of the condition or as a response to intervention. Since most conditions are likely to change over time, ongoing assessment is paramount to the appropriate selection of intervention. The types of measurement used in evaluating the response to treatment must be appropriate to the problems identified. The reader is referred to Chapter 1 for a full discussion of these issues.

References

1. Tortora G.J., Anagnostakos N.P. (1984). *Principles of Anatomy and Physiology* 4th edn. New York: Harper Row.
2. Oberholzer R.J.H., Tofani W.O. (1960). Neurophysiology. In *Handbook of Physiology* Vol. 2. American Physiological Society Press.
3. Goldman M.D. (1982). Interpretation of thoracoabdominal movement during breathing. *Clin. Sci.*, **62**, 7.
4. De Troyer A., Estenne M. (1984). Co-ordination between ribcage muscles and diaphragm during quiet breathing in humans. *J. Appl. Physiol.: Respirat. Environ. Exercise Physiol.*, **57**, 899.
5. De Troyer A., Sampson M.G. (1982). Activation of the parasternal intercostals during breathing efforts in human subjects. *J. Appl. Physiol.: Respirat. Environ. Exercise Physiol.*, **52**, 524.
6. Shaffer T.H., Wolfson M.R., Bhutani V.K. (1981). Respiratory muscle function, assessment and training. *Phys. Ther.*, **61**, 1711.

7. De Troyer A. (1984). Actions of the respiratory muscles, or how the chest wall moves in upright man. *Bull. Europ. Physiopath. Resp.*, **20**, 409.
8. Ellis E.R., Grunstein R.R., Chan S., *et al*. (1988). Non-invasive ventilative support during sleep reverses respiratory failure in kyphoscoliosis. *Chest*, **94**, 811.
9. White A.A., Panjabi M.M. (1978). *Clinical Biomechanics of the Spine.* Philadelphia: J.B. Lippincott, pp. 345–372.
10. Ellis E.R., McCauley V.B., Mellis C., *et al*. (1987). Treatment of alveolar hypoventilation in a six year old girl with IPPV through a nose mask. *Am. Rev. Respir. Dis.*, **136**, 188.
11. Fowler A.A., Scoggins W.G., O'Donohue W.J. (1978). Positive end-expiratory pressure in the management of lobar atelectasis. *Chest*, **74**, 497.
12. Britton S., Bejstedt M., Vedin L. (1985). Chest physiotherapy in primary pneumonia. *Br. Med. J.*, **290**, 1703.
13. Graham W.G.B., Bradely D.A. (1978). Efficacy of chest physiotherapy and intermittent positive pressure breathing in the resolution of pneumonia. *N. Engl. J. Med.*, **299**, 624–627.
14. Loring S.H., De Troyer A. (1985). Actions of the respiratory muscles. In *The Thorax* part A (Roussos C., Macklem P.T., eds.). New York: Marcel Dekker.
15. Ford G.T., Grant D.A., Rideout K.A., *et al*. (1988). Inhibition of breathing associated with gallbladder stimulation in dogs. *J. Appl. Physiol.*, **65**, 72.
16. Simmonneau G., Vivien A., Sartene R., *et al*. (1983). Diaphragm dysfunction induced by upper abdominal surgery – the role of postoperative pain. *Am. Rev. Respir. Dis.*, **128**, 899.
17. Ford G.T., Whitelaw W.A., Rosenal T.W., *et al*. (1983). Diaphragm function after upper abdominal surgery in humans. *Am. Rev. Respir. Dis.*, **127**, 431.
18. Dureuil B., Viires N., Cantineau J-P., *et al*. (1986). Diaphragm contractility after upper abdominal surgery. *J. Appl. Physiol.*, **61**, 1775.
19. Roussos C.S., Fixley M., Genest J., *et al*. (1977). Voluntary factors influencing the distribution of inspired gas. *Am. Rev. Respir. Dis.*, **116**, 457.
20. Larson V.H., Iverson A.D., Christensen P., *et al* (1985). Postoperative pain treatment after upper abdominal surgery with epidural morphine at thoracic or lumbar level. *Acta Anaesthesiol. Scand.*, **29**, 566.
21. Gottfried S., DiMarco A.F. (1989). Effect of intestinal afferent stimulation on pattern of respiratory muscle activation. *J. Appl. Physiol.*, **66** (3), 1455.
22. Hoover C.F. (1920). Diagnostic significance of inspiratory movements of costal margins. *Am. J. Med. Sci.*, **159**, 633.
23. Snider G.L. (1986). Chronic obstructive pulmonary disease – a continuing challenge. *Am. Rev. Respir. Dis.*, **133**, 942.
24. Farkas G.A., Roussos C. (1982). Adaptability of the hamster diaphragm to exercise and/or emphysema. *J. Appl. Physiol.*, **53**, 1263.
25. Braun N.M.T., Rochester D. (1977). Respiratory muscle function in chronic obstructive pulmonary disease (abstract). *Am. Rev. Respir. Dis.*, **115**, 91.
26. Macklem P.T. (1984). Hyperinflation. *Am. Rev. Respir. Dis.*, **129**, 1.
27. Luce J.M., Culver B.H. (1982). Respiratory muscle function in health and disease. *Chest*, **81**, 82.
28. Gilmartin J.J., Gibson G.J. (1984). Abnormalities of chest wall motion in patients with chronic airflow limitation. *Thorax*, **39**, 264.
29. Skarvan K., Mikalenka V. (1970). The ventilatory function of sternomastoid and scalene muscles in patients with pulmonary emphysema. *Respiration*, **27**, 480.
30. McCauley V., Grunstein R.R., Sullivan C.E. (1988). Ethanol-induced depression of hypoxic drive and reversal by naloxone – a sex difference. *Am. Rev. Respir. Dis.*, **137**, 1406.

31. Barach A.L., Beck G.J. (1954). The ventilatory effects of the head down position in pulmonary emphysema. *Am. J. Med.*, **26**, 55.
32. Barach A.L. (1974). Chronic obstructive lung disease: postural relief of dyspnoea. *Arch. Phys. Med. Rehabil.*, **55**, 494.
33. Sharp J.T., Druz W.S., Moisan T., *et al.* (1980). Postural relief of dyspnoea in severe chronic obstructive pulmonary disease. *Am. Rev. Respir. Dis.*, **122**, 201.
34. Higgs J., Wettenhall A.P. (1985). Designing a pulmonary rehabilitation programme. *Aust. J. Phys.*, **31**, 46.
35. Guyatt G.H., Berman L.B., Townsend M. (1987). Long term outcome after respiratory rehabilitation. *Can. Med. Assoc. J.*, **137**, 1089.
36. Ries A.L., Ellis B., Hawkins R.W. (1988). Upper extremity exercise training in chronic obstructive pulmonary disease. *Chest*, **93**, 688.
37. Carter R., Nicotra B., Clarke A., *et al.* (1988). Exercise conditioning in the rehabilitation of patients with chronic obstructive pulmonary disease. *Arch. Phys. Med. Rehabil.*, **69**, 118.
38. Levine S., Weiser P., Gillen J. (1986). Evaluation of ventilatory muscle endurance training in the rehabilitation of patients with chronic obstructive pulmonary disease. *Am. Rev. Respir. Dis.*, **133**, 400.
39. Larson J.L., Kim M.J., Sharp J.T., *et al.* (1988). Inspiratory muscle training with a pressure threshold device in patients with chronic obstructive pulmonary disease. *Am. Rev. Respir. Dis.*, **138**, 689.
40. Richardson J., Dunn L., Pardy R. (1989). Inspiratory resistive endurance training in patients with chronic obstructive pulmonary disease: a pilot study. *Phys. Can.*, **41**, 85.

Chapter 6

Mucociliary Clearance

JENNIFER PRYOR

INTRODUCTION

Mucociliary clearance is one of the means by which the lungs and the body are protected from particles inhaled on to the tracheobronchial mucosa. It involves two processes: first, the particles are trapped by the sticky mucous lining of the airways and secondly, they are transported out of the lungs by cilial action.

The walls of the trachea and bronchi comprise the mucosa, submucosa and a fibrocartilaginous and muscle layer. The mucosa is a pseudostratified, ciliated columnar epithelium containing numerous goblet cells (mucous cells). The epithelium decreases in thickness as the airways become smaller and it consists of a single layer of cuboid cells in the terminal bronchioli. In the respiratory bronchioli the ciliated epithelium becomes so thin that it is continuous with the alveolar ducts and alveoli. The alveolar epithelium comprises a layer of non-ciliated squamous cells. The goblet cells rest on a

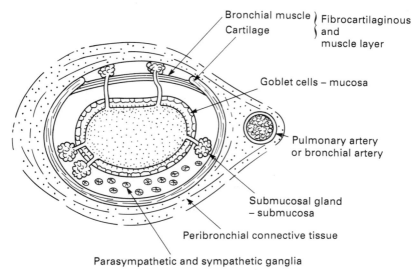

Figure 6.1   Cross-sectional diagrammatic representation of a large bronchus.

105

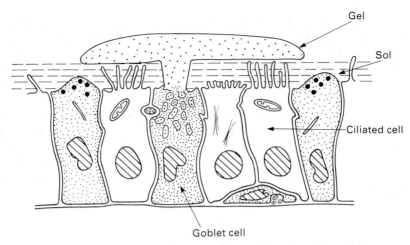

Figure 6.2   Cross-sectional diagrammatic representation of the mucosal layer of the airway.

basement membrane with submucosal glands containing mucus and serous elements lying in the submucosa (Figure 6.1).

Mucus is produced by the goblet cells and submucosal glands and is a complex substance consisting of water, glycoproteins, serum transudate, proteolytic enzymes and their inhibitors, locally produced immunoglobulins and lipids.[1] The pH is usually neutral. Secretion from the goblet cells is stimulated by irritation of the cells and secretion from the submucosal glands is stimulated by a vagal reflex and possibly by direct irritation. Local release of chemical mediators may also play a part. Airway mucus is a gel with special visco-elastic properties assisting propulsion by the respiratory cilia. As far back as 1934 a two-layer concept of respiratory mucus was documented.[2] The cilia are said to be surrounded by a watery periciliary fluid layer (sol) probably derived from transudation from the cells and covered by a mucous layer (gel) which interacts with the tips of the cilia. It is now thought that the mucous layer is discontinuous with foci of mucous droplets, desquamated cells, macrophages and cellular debris as opposed to a continuous mucous blanket (Figure 6.2).[3]

Mucociliary clearance in the small airways is slower than in the large airways.[4] This may be due to the reduction in cilial activity. The mechanisms involved in the movement of particles and macrophages from the alveolus to the bronchiolar ciliated epithelium are still hypothetical. The cilia extend from the ciliary cells of the mucous membrane and are about six micron in length. There are about 200 cilia per cell and 1500–2000 million/cm². Studies of the ultrastructure of cilia demonstrate a cilial shaft with nine pairs of filaments positioned circumferentially around a central pair of filaments (Figure 6.3). There are projections from each outer pair of filaments known as dynein arms. These arms or spokes are thought to coordinate ciliary bending and play an active part in maintaining effective ciliary beating. A rapid forward movement with a rigid cilium is followed by a slower recovery movement with a limp cilium (Figure 6.4). The cilia beat 360–960 times a minute and as they beat in succession a wave motion is produced. Ciliary movement must be coordinated to produce a propulsive wave for effective mucous clearance. There are hooks at the tips of the cilia which may increase the effectiveness of mucous transport. The rate of movement of the foci of mucus is said to be 2.5–33 mm per minute with smaller particles being carried faster than larger ones.

The ciliary escalator is continuous from the respiratory bronchioles to the trachea. Its efficiency depends on proper functioning of the cilia, the periciliary fluid and optimal thickness and visco-elasticity of the foci of mucus resting on the tips of the cilia. The relationship between viscosity and elasticity of the mucus probably has an effect on mucociliary clearance, but this has yet to be proven.

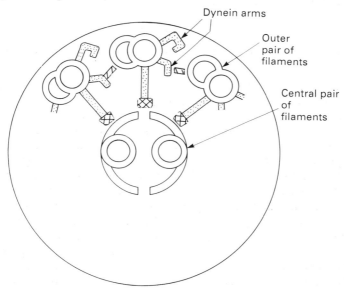

Figure 6.3 Cross-sectional diagrammatic representation of a cilium.

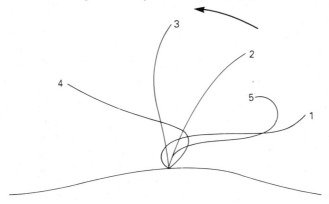

Figure 6.4 The movement of a cilium (1–5).

ABNORMAL MUCOCILIARY CLEARANCE

When mucociliary clearance is abnormal it is often difficult to determine which component is defective. If the mechanism is inadequate, coughing may augment mucus clearance. When the mucociliary escalator is functioning normally and the amount of mucus is not excessive, the clearance of mucus from the lungs is achieved by swallowing. Factors which can alter mucociliary clearance are: age, posture, sleep, mobility and exercise, environmental pollutants, disease, pharmacological agents, temperature and humidity,[4,5] hypoxia and hypercapnia[3]. Table 6.1 summarizes the information known to date.

In primary ciliary dyskinesia, the dynein arms are deficient in the cilia, producing defective ciliary beating. Ciliary dysfunction may also be activated by the sol.[1] Inhibition of the beating of human bronchial cilia, when exposed to the sol from the sputum of acute asthma, has been demonstrated. This effect diminishes or disappears as the asthma improves and may explain the decrease in mucociliary clearance during acute asthma.

TABLE 6.1
Factors affecting Mucociliary Clearance

Factors	Effect on Mucociliary Clearance
Age	Reduction in the elderly.[4]
Postural drainage	Increased in cystic fibrosis but not in normal subjects.[4]
Sleep	Reduction in both normal subjects and in asthmatics.[4]
Mobility and exercise	Increased with vigorous intensity exercise. Not affected by low intensity exercise such as daily activities.[4]
Environmental pollutants	Various effects on mucociliary clearance in studies relating to sulphur dioxide, tobacco smoke, ozone and fluorocarbon propellants, for example as in hair spray.[4]
Disease	Reduction in chronic bronchitis, asthma, bronchiectasis, viral, bacterial and mycoplasmal infections, immunoglobulin deficiency, pulmonary tuberculosis, bronchogenic carcinoma and primary ciliary dyskinesia (immotile cilia syndrome).[5]
Pharmacological agents	Probably increased by bromhexine, water, normal saline, hypertonic saline, beta-adrenergic drugs, theophyllines, corticosteroids and cholinergics. Unaltered or reduced by acetylcysteine, sodium cromoglycate, aspirin and anticholinergics (ipratropium bromide). Reduced by the inhalation of high oxygen (e.g. 90–100%), and anaesthetic agents.[4]
Dry cold air	Reduces mucociliary clearance, for example, when an artificial airway is present. The optimal temperature for cilia is normal body temperature (37°C).[4]
Hypoxia and hypercapnia	Reduction in mucociliary clearance.[3]
Commercially produced ionizers	Probably have no effect.

Sputum sol from bronchiectasis, with purulent sputum, has been shown to be toxic to human cilia, but when treated with antibiotics it is less toxic. Furthermore, bacteria are known to produce factors which are toxic to cilia. Infected mucus may damage the ciliated epithelium and there may be squamous metaplasia and consequent scarring of the airways. All these factors will contribute to decreased mucociliary clearance.

Signs and symptoms associated with problems of mucociliary clearance may occur singly or in combination and may be a direct or indirect result of these problems. They are found in association with various types of chest disease. The relationships between the functional disorder of impaired mucociliary clearance, the pathophysiology and presenting signs and symptoms are demonstrated in Figure 6.5.

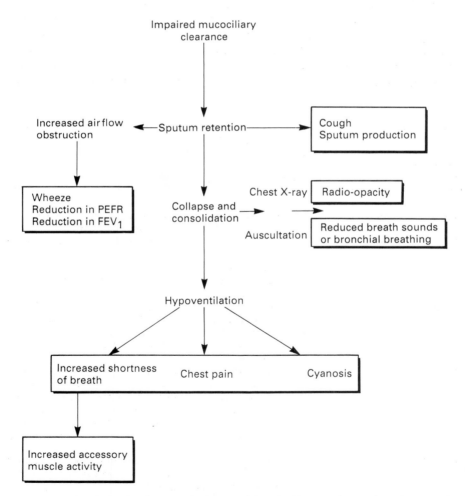

Figure 6.5 *The relationships between the functional disorder of impaired mucociliary clearance, the pathophysiology and the presenting signs and symptoms. Signs and symptoms are shown in boxes.*

TECHNIQUES FOR MUCOCILIARY CLEARANCE

Gravity

In the early 1900s a technique of 'empty bronchus treatment by posture in the bronchiectasis of children' was documented. This was continuous drainage and maintained for hours at a time. Later Nelson advocated intermittent posturing.[6] Individual drainage positions for specific bronchi became recognized and in 1956 a physiotherapist, Winifred Thacker, published a book *Postural Drainage* showing how the varying areas of the lung and air passages could be drained to the maximum advantage.[7] The positions were based on the anatomy of the bronchial tree. See Appendix B for specific drainage positions.

The specific positioning of the airways to allow gravity to assist the drainage and mobilization of excess bronchial secretions has long been accepted, but only recently has it been scientifically evaluated. Sutton and colleagues[8] showed that more sputum was expectorated when gravity-assisted positions were used. Hofmeyr and colleagues[9] also demonstrated that gravity-assisted positions increase sputum production when compared with that obtained from the sitting position alone. In these two studies gravity increased the efficiency of mucociliary clearance as measured by the amount of sputum being expectorated in a given time when combined with breathing techniques including thoracic expansion exercises, the forced expiration technique and breathing control.

For a lung segment which is productive of sputum, a minimum time of 10 minutes is recommended.[10] It is important to avoid treating more than two or three positions in the one treatment as treatment regimens covering several positions with four to five minutes in each position have been shown to cause a fall in transcutaneous oxygen tension.[11] It should be appreciated that the anatomical positions of the segments of the lung may alter with disease, for example pulmonary fibrosis, and will alter after pulmonary surgery, in particular resection of lung segments. In some subjects, when secretions are minimal, gravity-assisted positions may not be essential and breathing exercises in the sitting position alone may be as effective.

Percussion

The transmission of mechanical energy through the chest wall to the airways and consequent increase in intrathoracic pressure is generally considered to loosen excess bronchial secretions and to aid the clearance of these secretions. Percussion may be manual (chest clapping) or mechanical. Chest clapping, performed with a cupped hand and a relaxed flexion and extension of the wrists (Figure 6.6), has become the hallmark of the chest physiotherapist. Chest clapping is not intended to stimulate the skin and should be

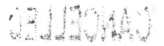

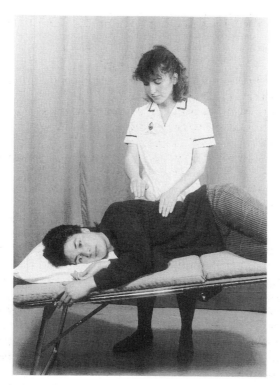

Figure 6.6 Chest clapping.

performed over clothes or a towel. In the surgical patient it is uncomfortable and should only be used when absolutely indicated. Chest clapping may be used to stimulate coughing in children under three years, who are unable to participate in the active cycle of breathing techniques.[10]

In patients with stable chronic chest disease and excess bronchial secretions there is no evidence to show that chest clapping alone will increase mucociliary clearance[12] or the expectoration of sputum.[13] Studies have yet to be done with patients in the acute phase of a bronchopulmonary infection. Chest clapping combined with other techniques and in the presence of an ineffective cough and very limited respiratory function, may be of value. Chest clapping has been shown both to decrease FEV_1[14] and to increase FVC.[15] It has also been shown to cause hypoxia,[16] but this can be prevented when chest clapping is combined with thoracic expansion exercises.[17]

Mechanical percussion may be applied externally[18] (Figure 6.7) or internally, for example, by using an oral high frequency oscillator (Figure

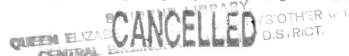

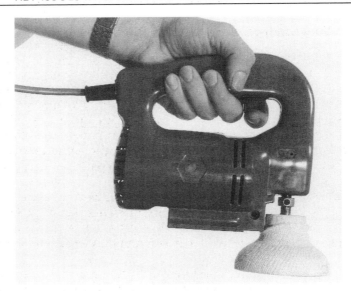

Figure 6.7 Mechanical percussor. (The Salford Percussor.)

6.8). Oral high frequency oscillation (OHFO) is the oscillation of the air within the airways at frequencies exceeding those of normal breathing. When external mechanical percussion was compared with chest clapping there was no significant difference in the weight of sputum expectorated.[19] OHFO may enhance mucociliary clearance,[20] but these studies were in normal people under laboratory conditions and studies of a wider range of conditions are necessary to support this evidence.

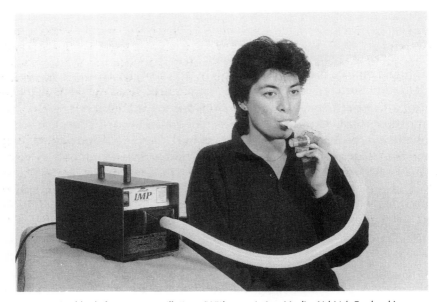

Figure 6.8 Oral high frequency oscillation. (With permission Medic-Aid Ltd, England.)

Chest Vibration, Chest Shaking and Chest Compression

The techniques of manual vibration, shaking or compression (squeezing) of the chest wall during an expiration will augment the expiratory flow rate. This may aid mucociliary clearance, but studies of these techniques are not yet available. Chest vibration, shaking and/or compression may be done by an assistant (Figure 6.9) or by the individual (Figure 6.10). For these techniques the hands are placed over the appropriate part of the chest wall along the line of the ribs. The hands follow the natural movement of the chest wall. Care must be taken where there is pain, a fracture or osteoporosis.

Vibration is a fine, rapidly oscillating movement of the chest wall. The fingers and the palm of the hand are in contact with the chest wall although most of the vibration force is exerted through the fingers. Care must be taken not to exert uncomfortable pressure with the tips of the fingers.

Shaking is a large amplitude, vigorous movement of the chest wall. The whole hand is in contact with the chest wall although most of the pressure is exerted through the palm.

Compression is where the therapist applies a relatively constant compressive force to the chest wall to assist the individual to increase the expiratory force. Compression can be used in combination with other techniques such as the forced expiration technique and can be used by the individuals themselves.

Cough

The function of the cough is to remove foreign material and secretions from the upper airways. Under normal circumstances we cough infrequently and the mucociliary escalator is an effective clearance mechanism on its own. The cough becomes a powerful, supplementary clearance mechanism for the rapid removal of foreign particles. It is also important in diseases in which there are changes in the quality and quantity of bronchial mucus and changes in airway structure.

Coughing is most effective at high expiratory flows and it is at high lung volumes that these high flows are achieved.[21] A cough may be initiated voluntarily or may be reflex. A deep inspiration is followed by closure of the glottis, and contraction of the muscles of the chest wall and abdomen increase the subglottic pressure. The glottis suddenly opens and expiratory flows may exceed 120 metres per second[22] expelling excess secretions and particulate matter.

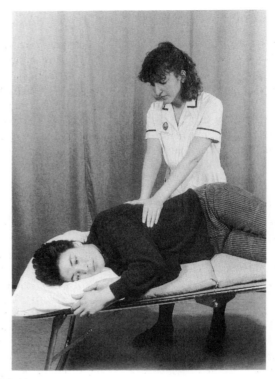

Figure 6.9   Chest shaking.

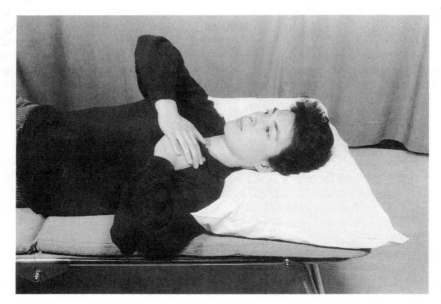

Figure 6.10   Self compression.

Panting*

For people who cannot cough effectively, sputum removal from upper airways can also be encouraged with a manoeuvre called panting. The person is instructed to take four or five shallow breaths at a high lung volume maintaining an even rate and tidal volume. The breaths should be in rapid succession with an emphasis on expiration. Compression can be added by the therapist on expiration to enhance the expiratory effort. Often this manoeuvre will trigger a cough in those who cannot generate one voluntarily. In addition, the manoeuvre appears to move secretions up the airway to a point where the patient can clear them easily without coughing.

Thoracic Expansion Exercises

The alternating shortening and narrowing, and lengthening and widening of the bronchial tree, during expiration and inspiration has a 'milking' effect on the mucous blanket and its particulate matter. This effect can be augmented by deep breathing exercises also known as thoracic expansion exercises. Deep breathing, in addition, may bring in alternative pathways for airflow. The collateral ventilatory system[23] comprising the inter-alveolar, alveolar-bronchiole and inter-bronchiole channels (Figure 6.11) is thought to be the means by which air can be found distal to mucous plugs in the peripheral airways.

Another mechanism by which increasing tidal volume[24] can probably move air into small airways obstructed by secretions is the phenomenon of interdependence.[25] During inspiration, expanding alveoli exert a force on adjacent alveoli. This force is referred to as interdependence and may aid in the re-expansion of collapsed alveoli. The effects of interdependence and collateral ventilation are said to be more marked during deep breathing. Postoperatively the use of thoracic expansion exercises with a three-second hold at the end of inspiration has been shown to decrease atelectasis.[26] In many chronic lung diseases where there is already a degree of hyperinflation the three second hold may not be indicated.

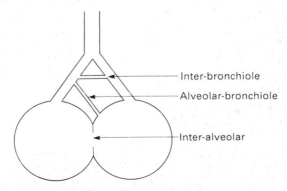

Inter-bronchiole

Alveolar-bronchiole

Inter-alveolar

Figure 6.11 The collateral ventilatory system.

* This technique has been included at the request of the volume editors.

The Forced Expiration Technique

The forced expiration technique (FET) is one or two **huffs or forced expirations, combined with breathing control.** During a forced expiration (huff or cough), compressive forces occurring within the airways move down the airways (towards the alveoli) as lung volume decreases. The point at which compression occurs is referred to as the equal pressure point[27] and the dynamic compression which takes place downstream (towards the mouth) of the equal pressure point is an essential part of the clearance mechanism. The intrathoracic pressures generated with huffing are not as high as with coughing which can be an advantage when a patient is in pain or has particularly collapsible airways. To produce a huff, a breath is taken in and, using the abdominal and chest muscles, the air is squeezed out while keeping the mouth open. It is necessary to continue the huff down to low lung volumes when the aim is to clear secretions from the more peripheral airways. A huff from a high lung volume will dislodge secretions from the upper airways, for example the trachea. This is sometimes known as a huff cough.

When difficulties are encountered in producing an effective huff,[28] blowing down a peak expiratory flow meter mouth piece, huffing or blowing pieces of paper are techniques which can be used. Children, from the age of two or three years, can be introduced to huffing games.[29]

Breathing control is gentle breathing using the lower chest with relaxation of the upper chest and shoulders. This was known as diaphragmatic breathing, but as there is well documented activity of the intercostal muscles, the abdominal muscles and the scalene muscles while breathing at rest,[30] breathing control has replaced the term diaphragmatic breathing.[10]

The FET is usually used as a part of the active cycle of breathing techniques in postural drainage positions or in sitting. The regimen is adapted to suit the individual patient and an example of the cycle is as follows:

1 Breathing control
2 Three or four thoracic expansion exercises with or without chest clapping
3 Breathing control
4 One or two thoracic expansion exercises with or without chest shaking
5 Breathing control
6 One or two huffs with or without chest compression } FET
7 Breathing control

The cycle is repeated until secretions are no longer being expectorated or the patient requires a rest. A minimum of ten minutes is recommended for a position which is producing a significant amount of sputum. A postural drainage regimen including the FET may be used with or without an assistant.

If thoracic expansion exercises are not included with the periods of chest clapping and if the periods of breathing control are omitted, a fall in oxygen saturation may result.[16] The use of the FET and the active cycle of breathing techniques can prevent this hypoxaemia.[17]

The use of FET has been shown to be an effective means of mobilizing and expectorating excess bronchial secretions without increasing airflow obstruction.[31] It has also been shown to improve pulmonary function.[32]

Autogenic Drainage

Autogenic drainage (AD) is the use of breathing control and thoracic expansion exercises, at varying lung volumes, to obtain maximal expiratory flow in the different generations of bronchi. Studies of iso-volume flow loops demonstrate higher flows with unforced rather than forced expiratory manoeuvres,[33] but this phenomenon exists only in subjects with pressure dependent airway collapse. It is claimed that mucus within the airways is moved further and at a faster rate using these higher flows, but this has not been proven.

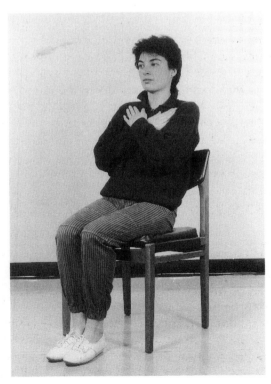

Figure 6.12   Position for autogenic drainage.

Autogenic drainage is performed sitting upright, relaxed, with the neck slightly extended and the hands placed over the upper part of the thorax (Figure 6.12). The phases of autogenic drainage are said to be 'unstick', 'collect' and 'evacuate'.[33] Mucus in the peripheral lung regions is usually mobilized first using breathing control, at a low lung volume. The more central regions require breathing control at a high lung volume. The level at which the mucus is situated is assessed and the level of ventilated volume required to mobilize it is then selected. The time factor is a disadvantage as a treatment session takes about an hour.

Positive Airway Pressure Devices

The **Positive Expiratory Pressure** (PEP) mask provides positive expiratory pressure during expiration. This is said to prevent airways from collapsing and to allow air to move behind mucous plugs by utilizing the collateral ventilatory system.[11] It is advocated that the PEP mask be used in the sitting position with the arms resting comfortably on a table (Figure 6.13). The mask has a one-way valve to which expiratory resistances can be attached. It is held tightly over the nose and mouth. Lower chest breathing is used with a slightly active expiration. A pressure of 12–17 cmH$_2$O in the middle third of

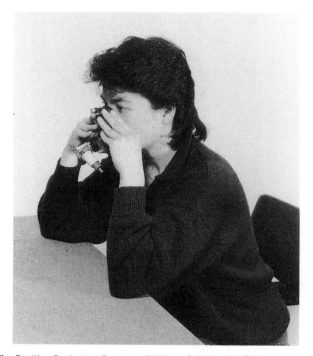

Figure 6.13 The Positive Expiratory Pressure (PEP) mask (Astra Meditec)

expiration is recommended and this is achieved by selecting the appropriate expiratory resistance. Six to twelve breaths are followed by forced expirations and breathing control and the cycle is repeated for 15 minutes. A study which looked at the PEP mask as an adjunct to the postural drainage regimen using the FET and the active cycle of breathing techniques,[9] did not demonstrate an advantage in the clearance of bronchial secretions when PEP was used. The gravity-assisted positions with and without PEP produced more sputum than PEP in the sitting position alone.

Intermittent Positive Pressure Breathing (IPPB) is the maintenance of a positive pressure, within the airways, throughout inspiration. It is often administered by a pressure cycled ventilator (Figure 6.14). IPPB can reduce the work of breathing[34] and can increase tidal volume.[35] It has been used as a mechanical adjunct in the treatment of respiratory failure.[36] A study concluded that IPPB can be used as an alternative to chest physiotherapy in sputum-producing patients where the active cycle of breathing techniques is not possible.[37] When sufficient expiratory flows cannot be generated voluntarily to aid effective mucociliary clearance IPPB may be of assistance. IPPB may be used when a patient has excess bronchial secretions in the presence

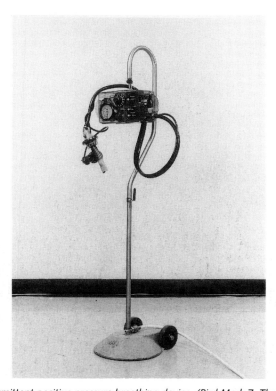

Figure 6.14   Intermittent positive pressure breathing device. (Bird Mark 7. The Bird Corporation.)

of respiratory fatigue, cerebral injury, mental confusion or the inability to respond to verbal instructions, chest wall deformity or marked respiratory muscle weakness.

IPPB can be useful integrated with other physiotherapy techniques for mucociliary clearance such as gravity-assisted positioning, thoracic expansion exercises and the forced expiration technique. As a means of administering bronchodilators, IPPB is probably no more effective than the continuous flow nebulizer[38] or the metered dose inhaler.[39]

The literature evaluating IPPB is conflicting. Studies show increases and decreases in ventilation and in the work of breathing, improvements and deteriorations in blood gases, with the user feeling subjectively worse or better. These differences may be due to the skill of the therapist, as the technique of using IPPB may alter its effectiveness. Careful instruction and knowledge of the contraindications is essential. Contraindications to positive airway pressure include pneumothorax, bullae, lung abscess, post-operative air leaks and bronchial tumour in the proximal airways.

Periodic Continuous Positive Airway Pressure (PCPAP) is the periodic use of a positive pressure, within the airways, throughout inspiration and expiration, in the spontaneously breathing patient (Figure 6.15). The source

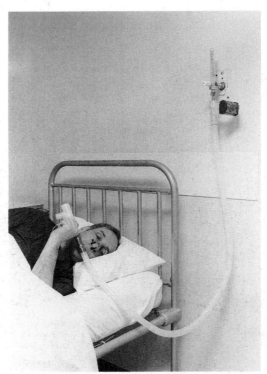

Figure 6.15   PCPAP in side-lying. (Reproduced from Webber B.A. The Brompton Hospital Guide to Chest Physiotherapy. 5th edn. London: Blackwell Scientific Publications. With permission The Brompton Hospital © 1988.)

of the positive pressure is a high flow generator and PCPAP is administe
via a mask or a mouthpiece and nose clip. In clinical practice, a pressure
5–10 cmH$_2$O is produced by means of a positive end expiratory pressure
valve.

PCPAP reduces the work of breathing and increases functional residual
capacity.[40] The increase in functional residual capacity (FRC) aids mucociliary clearance by improving collateral ventilation, by the phenomenon of
interdependence and by reducing the resistance of obstructed airways.
Re-expansion of areas of atelectasis will also increase mucociliary clearance.
It is known that FEV$_1$, FVC and FRC are reduced, postoperatively, for up to
14 days.[41] The decrease in FRC may be the most important factor leading to
small airway closure and decreased mucociliary clearance. The effect of
increasing FRC using PCPAP makes it a useful adjunct in the treatment of
postoperative pulmonary complications[42] and in the mobilization of excess
bronchial secretions in medical chest conditions.

PCPAP can be used in sitting or in a postural drainage or modified
postural drainage position. A period of CPAP is given for 10 to 15 minutes
and this can be followed by the active cycle of breathing techniques including thoracic expansion exercises and the forced expiration technique.
Chest clapping is usually omitted as it may reduce FRC[11] and negate the
effect of the PCPAP.

Incentive spirometry

An incentive spirometer is a device which provides some feedback to
the patient of either inspiratory flow rate or tidal volume. An incentive

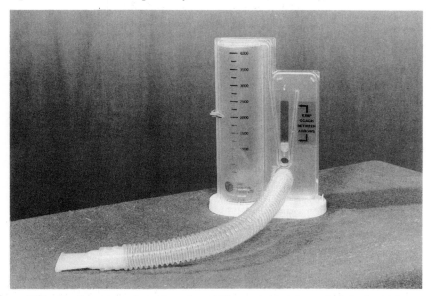

Figure 6.16   The Coach incentive spirometer. (With permission Intersurgical, England.)

spirometer used effectively is an alternative for providing motivation for thoracic expansion exercises, probably utilizing collateral ventilation, interdependence and reducing the resistance to airflow by increasing lung volume (Figure 6.16). A volume-dependent rather than flow-dependent device should be used for maximal effect to be obtained. A deep breath with a 3-second hold produces the same effect. Studies[43,44] have concluded that deep breathing exercises are as effective as incentive spirometry in preventing postoperative pulmonary complications and consequently in maintaining or increasing mucociliary clearance. Incentive spirometry provides some motivation for deep breathing exercises with an inspiratory hold, in children, adolescents and adults experiencing difficulty in changing their pattern of breathing voluntarily.

Humidification and Nebulization

When breathing through the nose or mouth, the inspired air is warmed and humidified. The air is fully saturated and at a temperature of 37°C by the time it reaches the trachea. If a person is required to breathe dry gases for any length of time, this will tend to dry out the mucosa of the upper

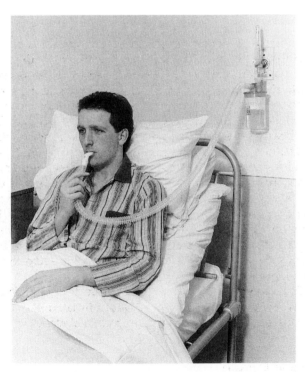

Figure 6.17   Humidification from a large volume nebulizer. (Reproduced from Webber B.A. The Brompton Hospital Guide to Chest Physiotherapy. 5th edn. London: Blackwell Scientific Publications. With permission The Brompton Hospital © 1988.)

respiratory tract. High humidity or additional water content can be provided by humidifiers, nebulizers or a combination of the two. A **humidifier** (Figure 6.17) is a device which produces water vapour. A **nebulizer** utilizes the jet principle to break the water up into small particles or droplets suspended in a stream of gas. **Ultrasonic nebulizers** operate on the principle of high-frequency sound waves passing through a solution and producing an aerosol. Both humidifers and nebulizers can be heated to increase the degree of humidity. Deposition of these droplets within the airways depends on their size, the pattern of breathing and on the degree of airflow obstruction. Particles with a mass median aerodynamic diameter of less than 5µ can be peripherally deposited. Particles above 5µ are more likely to be deposited in the upper respiratory tract.[10] These larger particles may facilitate the expectoration of sputum.

Water and normal saline (0.9%) are used for humidification and Sutton and colleagues[45] have shown an increase in mucociliary clearance when postural drainage together with FET is preceded by five minutes inhalation of nebulized normal saline. Nebulized hypertonic saline (7.0%) can also increase mucociliary clearance.[46]

Drugs

Drugs can influence mucociliary clearance by stimulating cilial activity, through bronchodilatation or by altering the viscosity of the mucus. Drugs which can increase cilial activity include some of the beta-adrenergic agents such as salbutamol[47] and terbutaline.[48] As bacteria can have a toxic effect on cilia, appropriate antibiotics may increase mucociliary clearance. To aid mucociliary clearance, maximal bronchodilatation should be achieved before other clearance techniques are used. Beta-adrenergic drugs such as salbutamol, fenoterol, terbutaline and anticholinergic agents such as ipratropium bromide are known bronchodilators. Mucolytic agents, for example acetylcysteine, are used, supposedly to reduce the viscosity of the bronchial secretions. There is no evidence however, to support an increase in mucociliary clearance following the inhalation of these agents and they may increase airflow obstruction. Mucociliary clearance may be more affected by alterations in elasticity rather than viscosity of the mucus. It may be more difficult for the ciliary escalator to move fluid, watery secretions than secretions which are more viscid.

Drugs such as bronchodilators, mucolytics and antibiotics can be taken either orally or by inhalation. The advantage of inhalation of these agents is that smaller doses can be used to obtain a maximal effect.

Ambulation and Exercise

Vigorous exercise, for example, swimming and static bicycle riding, has been shown to increase mucociliary clearance.[4] Short-term studies of exercise training programmes have demonstrated improvements in sputum clearance.[49] Exercise is beneficial in addition to the other techniques for mucociliary clearance, but it should not be used as a substitute.[49]

In a group of patients following coronary artery bypass graft surgery, early ambulation has been shown to be as effective as incentive spirometry in preventing postoperative pulmonary complications and decreased mucociliary clearance.[50] Ambulation would seem to increase mucociliary clearance and should be used in addition to the other techniques.

Glossopharyngeal Breathing

Glossopharyngeal breathing is a method of assisted coughing.[10] It is of value in paralysis of the respiratory muscles, for example, tetraplegia and poliomyelitis where there is a reduced vital capacity and an ineffective cough. Glossopharyngeal breathing augments vital capacity and leads to a more effective cough. It is a form of positive pressure breathing produced by the patient's voluntary muscles. A series of pumping strokes are performed, during inspiration, by the action of the lips, mouth, tongue, soft palate, pharynx and larynx. Air is held in by the larynx acting as an intermittent valve and expiration is passive. To produce a maximal vital capacity and an effective cough 10–20 gulps are required depending on the volume of each gulp. Glossopharyngeal breathing is a technique which may require time and patience to master, but it will increase mucociliary clearance in those with respiratory muscle paralysis. The technique may be combined with chest compression during the expiratory phase and may be used in gravity-assisted positions.

Pain Relief

When pain is present, measures taken to reduce or eliminate it will increase the effectiveness of the techniques used and increase mucociliary clearance. Physiotherapy will be more effective if timed to coincide with adequate analgesics. Alternatively, physical modalities including transcutaneous electrical nerve stimulation (TENS)[51] and the inhalation of Entonox[10] can be used with or as an alternative to, oral analgesic agents. Entonox is premixed oxygen (50%) and nitrous oxide (50%). It is an analgesic which has a rapidly induced effect, but does not persist for more than two to four minutes after the end of the inhalation. It can be used to provide short-term pain relief to cover the treatment period.

CASE STUDIES

Case Study 1

Assessment. Clinical History: A 20-year-old man with cystic fibrosis was admitted to hospital with an exacerbation of his bronchopulmonary infection. He had noticed increasing shortness of breath on exertion and increased sputum over the past month. **Physical Assessment:** On auscultation he had widespread crackles, most marked in his mid zones. His sputum was thick and purulent. His medical management included inhaled salbutamol four times a day and intravenous and inhaled antibiotics. **Clinical tests:** His chest X-ray showed widespread fibrotic shadowing throughout both lung fields. He was febrile. His FEV_1 was 0.50 litres (predicted normal: 3.70 litres) and FVC was 0.85 litres (predicted normal: 4.20 litres). He was referred to the physiotherapist.

Analysis

There appeared to be excessive bronchial secretions throughout both lung fields, in particular the middle lobe, lingula, anterior segments of the upper lobes and lateral segments of the lower lobes as evidenced by auscultation. In addition, he had decreased exercise tolerance as evidenced by the exercise testing and clinical history.

Treatment Plan

1 To improve mucociliary clearance by
    a adequate bronchodilator therapy;
    b by ensuring adequate humidification of secretions;
    c by postural drainage and sputum removal techniques.
2 To assess exercise tolerance using a progressive exercise test on a cycle ergometer when afebrile.
3 To improve exercise tolerance by using a progressive exercise programme based on the results of the exercise test.

Details of Treatment

1 Inhaled nebulized salbutamol was given as prescribed with normal saline, in the sitting position, timed for maximal bronchodilator effect during treatment.
2 Ten minutes of heated and nebulized normal saline, in the sitting position was given after the salbutamol and before postural drainage. The peak expiratory flow rate was recorded before and after humidity on the first occasion to ensure that high humidity did not increase airflow obstruction.
3 From an assessment using the chest X-ray, auscultation and clinical history the most productive positions were determined. Four treatment sessions were planned for each day: (1) lateral segments of the lower lobes, (2) anterior segments of the upper lobes, (3) right middle zone and lingula, (4) anterior segments of the upper lobes. The following techniques were chosen and continued until there was no longer any sputum produced in each drainage position:

Breathing control to prevent undue fatigue and hypoxia

3–4 thoracic expansion exercises with chest clapping to mobilize the secretions

Breathing control

1–2 huffs with chest shaking or chest compression to move the secretions proximally

Breathing control

When practical, the patient was encouraged to perform some of the treatment himself to establish independence and to prepare for ongoing management at home.

4 Inhaled nebulized antibiotics were given twice a day following the appropriate postural drainage session to ensure that as much antibiotic as possible was deposited in the lung.

5 60% of the maximum work load achieved was used as the starting point for exercise. Cycling was undertaken daily for a 15-minute period and the work load was increased gradually each day.

Evaluation and Recommendations

Treatment would be continued within each session until the cycle of breathing techniques no longer produced expectoration of sputum, unless the treatment was poorly tolerated and the patient should be given a rest. As the sputum decreases in quantity and purulence, the number of postural drainage sessions would be reduced and by discharge, on approximately the seventh day, two treatments would be carried out, one with assistance and one without. On discharge a postural drainage frame (Figure 6.18) may be provided for use in the home. Cycling would also be continued at home using a static bicycle.

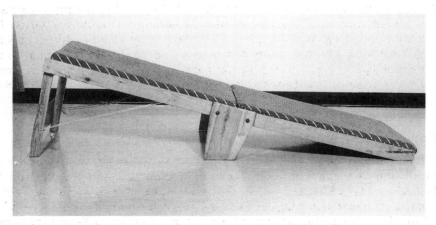

Figure 6.18 Postural drainage frame. (Reproduced from Webber B.A. The Brompton Hospital Guide to Chest Physiotherapy. 5th edn. London: Blackwell Scientific Publications. With permission The Brompton Hospital © 1988.)

Case Study 2

Assessment. Clinical History: A 55-year-old woman, obese and a known heavy smoker, became febrile on the second day following a hysterectomy. **Clinical Tests:** Her preoperative film had been clear; however her chest X-ray showed right lower lobe atelectasis postoperatively. **Physical Assessment:** She had a weak, dry sounding, non-productive cough and on auscultation bronchial breathing could be heard over the right lung base posteriorly.

Analysis

Because of the effects of surgery, in particular the abdominal pain, this person was unable to clear tenacious, bronchial secretions effectively. The pain from the wound inhibited the cough reflex and spontaneous deep breaths.

Treatment Plan

1 To reduce the effects of the pain.
2 To facilitate the removal of secretions without causing discomfort or exacerbating the airways closure.
3 To re-expand the right lower lobe atelectasis with periodic continuous positive airway pressure (PCPAP), with the right lower lobe placed in a non-dependent position.

Details of Treatment

1 Regular analgesics were taken orally as prescribed, prior to physiotherapy treatment.
2 Following a short time on PCPAP, in the left side lying position, her huff sounded crackly. The active cycle of breathing techniques (referred to earlier), omitting chest clapping, was followed by a further 10 minutes of PCPAP and the breathing techniques repeated. This regimen was repeated in sitting. She was encouraged to continue lower thoracic expansion exercises with a three second hold half hourly followed by one or two huffs.

Evaluation and Recommendations

If breath sounds at the right lung base were absent the treatment would need to be continued on a regular basis. Two hours later the regimen of PCPAP and breathing techniques would be repeated. Her huff should then become productive of plugs of thick, purulent sputum and breath sounds, although reduced, should become normal. A repeat chest X-ray may show expansion of the right lower lobe although some reduction in volume is likely to persist. The PCPAP regimen would be used four times the following day with breathing exercises continued during the waking hours. PCPAP would then be reduced to twice and the next day discontinued. By this time the huff and cough should become dry sounding and non-productive with the chest X-ray showing complete re-expansion of the right lower lobe. She should continue the breathing exercises, on her own, three times a day until discharge. Ambulation would be encouraged from the first post-operative day.

This chapter has examined the physiotherapy management of problems of mucociliary clearance. It is the physiotherapist's responsibility to re-evaluate the problems and analyse the response to treatment techniques. Testing of established known techniques and assessment of new techniques is an important part of the therapist's role. Chest physiotherapy is an applied science, however, we must not forget that its application is human.

ACKNOWLEDGEMENTS

I wish to thank Sonya Lam for her help with the figures, and Elizabeth Ellis and Jennifer Alison for their editorial assistance.

REFERENCES

1. Greenstone M., Cole P.J. (1985). Ciliary function in health and disease. *Br. J. Dis. Chest*, **79, 9**.
2. Lucas A.M., Douglas L.C. (1934). Principles underlying ciliary activity in the respiratory tract. *Arch. Otolaryngol.*, **20, 518**.
3. Wanner A. (1977). Clinical aspects of mucociliary transport. *Am. Rev. Respir. Dis.*, **116, 73**.
4. Pavia D. (1984). Lung mucociliary clearance. In *Aerosols and The Lung* (Clarke S.W., Pavia D, eds.). London: Butterworths, pp. 127–155.
5. Pavia D. (1987). Acute respiratory infections and mucociliary clearance. *Eur. J. Respir. Dis.* **71, 219**.
6. Nelson H.P. (1934). Postural drainage of the lungs. *Br. Med. J.*, **2, 251**.
7. Thacker E.W. (1956). *Postural Drainage*. London: Lloyd-Luke.
8. Sutton P.P., Parker R.A., Webber B.A., *et al.* (1983). Assessment of the forced expiration technique, postural drainage and directed coughing in chest physiotherapy. *Eur. J. Respir. Dis*, **64, 62**.
9. Hofmeyr J.L., Webber B.A., Hodson M.E. (1986). Evaluation of positive expiratory pressure as an adjunct to chest physiotherapy in the treatment of cystic fibrosis. *Thorax*, **41, 951**.
10. Webber B.A. (1988). *The Brompton Hospital Guide to Chest Physiotherapy* 5th edn. London: Blackwell Scientific Publications.
11. Falk M., Kelstrup M., Andersen J.B., *et al.* (1984). Improving the ketchup bottle method with positive expiratory pressure, PEP, in cystic fibrosis. *Eur. J. Respir. Dis*, **65, 423**.
12. van der Schans C.P., Piers D.A., Postma D.S. (1986). Effect of manual percussion on tracheobronchial clearance in patients with chronic airflow obstruction and excessive tracheobronchial secretion. *Thorax*, **41, 448**.

13. Webber B.A., Parker R.A. Hofmeyr J.L. *et al.* (1985). Evaluation of self-percussion during postural drainage using the forced expiration technique. *Physiotherapy Practice*, **1**, 42.
14. Campbell A.H., O'Connell J.M., Wilson F. (1975). The effect of chest physiotherapy upon the FEV_1 in chronic bronchitis. *Med. J. Aust.*, **1**, 33.
15. Tecklin J.S., Holsclaw D.S. (1975). Evaluation of bronchial drainage in patients with cystic fibrosis. *Phys. Ther.*, **55**, 1081.
16. McDonnell T., McNicholas W.T., Fitzgerald M.X. (1986). Hypoxaemia during chest physiotherapy in patients with cystic fibrosis. *Ir. J. Med. Sci.*, **155**, 345.
17. Pryor J.A., Webber B.A., Hodson M.E. (1990). Effect of chest physiotherapy on oxygen saturation in patients with cystic fibrosis. *Thorax*, **45**, 77.
18. Flower K.A., Eden R.I., Lomax L. *et al.* (1979). The new mechanical aid to physiotherapy in cystic fibrosis. *Br. Med. J.*, **2**, 630.
19. Pryor J.A., Parker R.A., Webber B.A. (1981). A comparison of mechanical and manual percussion as adjuncts to postural drainage in the treatment of cystic fibrosis in adolescents and adults. *Physiotherapy*, **67**, 140.
20. George R.J.D., Johnson M.A., Pavia D., *et al.* (1985). Increase in mucociliary clearance in normal man induced by oral high frequency oscillation. *Thorax*, **40**, 433.
21. Leith D. (1968). Cough. *Phys. Ther.*, **48**, 439.
22. Macklem P.T. (1974) Physiology of cough. *Transactions of the American Broncho-Esophalogical Association*, pp. 150–157.
23. Menkes H.A., Traystman R.J. (1977). Collateral ventilation. *Am. Rev. Respir. Dis.*, **116**, 287.
24. Menkes H.A., Britt J. (1980). Rationale for physical therapy. *Am.Rev.Respir. Dis.*, **122** (Suppl. part 2) 127.
25. Mead J., Takishima T., Leith D. (1970). Stress distribution in lungs: a model of pulmonary elasticity. *J. Appl. Physiol.*, **28**, 596.
26. Ward R.J., Danziger F., Bonica J.J., *et al.* (1966). An evaluation of post-operative respiratory maneuvers. *Surg. Gynecol. Obstet.*, **123**, 51.
27. West J.B. (1985). *Respiratory Physiology – the Essentials* 3rd edn. Baltimore: Williams & Wilkins, pp. 105–108.
28. Partridge C., Pryor J., Webber B. (1989). Characteristics of the forced expiration technique. *Physiotherapy*, **75**, 193.
29. Thompson B. (1978). *Asthma and Your Child* 5th edn. Christchurch, New Zealand: Pegasus Press.
30. Green M., Moxham J. (1985). The respiratory muscles. *Clin. Sci.*, **68**, 1.
31. Pryor J.A., Webber B.A. (1979). An evaluation of the forced expiration technique as an adjunct to postural drainage. *Physiotherapy*, **65** (10), 304.
32. Webber B.A, Hofmeyr J.L., Morgan M.D.L., *et al.* (1986). Effects of postural drainage, incorporating the forced expiration technique, on pulmonary function in cystic fibrosis. *Br. J. Dis. Chest*, **80**, 353.
33. Schöni M.H. (1989). Autogenic drainage: a modern approach to physiotherapy in cystic fibrosis. *J. R. Soc. Med.*, **82** (Suppl. 16), 32.
34. Ayres S.M., Kozam R.L., Lucas D.S. (1963). The effects of intermittent positive pressure breathing on intrathoracic pressure, pulmonary mechanics and the work of breathing. *Am. Rev. Respir. Dis.*, **87**, 370.
35. Sukumalchantra Y., Park S.S., Williams M.H. (1965). The effect of intermittent positive pressure breathing (IPPB) in acute ventilatory failure. *Am. Rev. Respir. Dis.*, **92**, 885.
36. Starke I.D., Webber B.A., Branthwaite M.A. (1979). IPPB and hypercapnia in respiratory failure: the effect of different concentrations of inspired oxygen on arterial blood gas tensions. *Anaesthesia*, **34**, 283.

37. Pavia D., Webber B.A., Agnew J.E., *et al.* (1988). The role of intermittent positive pressure breathing (IPPB) in bronchial toilet. *Eur. Respir. J.*, **1** (Suppl. 2) 250S.
38. Webber B.A., Shenfield G.M., Paterson J.W. (1974). A comparison of three different techniques for giving nebulised albuterol to asthmatic patients. *Am. Rev. Respir. Dis.*, **109**, 293.
39. Cayton R.M., Webber B., Paterson, J.W. *et al.* (1978). A comparison of salbutamol given by pressure-packed aerosol or nebulization via IPPB in acute asthma. *Br. J. Dis. Chest*, **72**, 222.
40. Gherini S., Peters R.M., Virgilio R.W. (1979). Mechanical work on the lungs and work of breathing with positive end-expiratory pressure and continuous positive airway pressure. *Chest*, **76**, 251.
41. Craig D.B. (1981). Postoperative recovery of pulmonary function. *Anesth. Analg.*, **60**(1), 46.
42. Andersen J.B., Olesen K.P., Eikard B., *et al.* (1980). Periodic continuous positive airway pressure, CPAP, by mask in the treatment of atelectasis. *Eur. J. Respir. Dis.*, **61**, 20.
43. Celli B.R., Rodriguez K.S., Snider G.L. (1984). A controlled trial of intermittent positive pressure breathing, incentive spirometry, and deep breathing exercises in preventing pulmonary complications after abdominal surgery. *Am. Rev. Respir. Dis.*, **130**, 12.
44. Stock M.C., Downs J.B., Gauer P.K., *et al.* (1985). Prevention of postoperative pulmonary complications with CPAP, incentive spirometry and conservative therapy. *Chest*, **87**, 151.
45. Sutton P.P., Gemmell H.G., Innes N., *et al.* (1988). Use of nebulised saline and nebulised terbutaline as an adjunct to chest physiotherapy. *Thorax*, **43**, 57.
46. Pavia D., Thomson M.L., Clarke S.W. (1978). Enhanced clearance of secretions from the human lung after the administration of hypertonic saline aerosol. *Am. Rev. Respir. Dis.*, **117**, 199.
47. Lafortuna C.L., Fazio F. (1984). Acute effect of inhaled salbutamol on mucociliary clearance in health and chronic bronchitis. *Respiration*, **45**, 111.
48. Wood R.E., Wanner A., Hirsch J., *et al.* (1975). Tracheal mucociliary transport in patients with cystic fibrosis and its stimulation by terbutaline. *Am. Rev. Respir. Dis.*, **111**, 733.
49. Dodd M.E. (1991). Exercise in cystic fibrosis adults. In *Respiratory Care* (Pryor J.A. ed.) Edinburgh: Churchill Livingstone, pp. 27–50.
50. Jenkins S.C., Soutar S.A., Loukota J.M., *et al.* (1989). Physiotherapy after coronary artery surgery: are breathing exercises necessary? *Thorax*, **44**, 634.
51. Mannheimer J.S. (1985). TENS: Uses and effectiveness. In *Pain* (Hoskins M.T. ed.). Edinburgh: Churchill Livingstone, pp. 73–121.

Chapter 7

Pulmonary Limitations to Exercise Performance

JENNIFER ALISON, ELIZABETH ELLIS

INTRODUCTION

No matter how sedentary a person's lifestyle, there is always the need to perform some exercise, be it walking to the station, making beds, climbing stairs or shopping. There are of course many jobs that require particularly strenuous activity, e.g., mining, brick-laying; and many recreational activities that require high levels of exertion, e.g., tennis, swimming, jogging, football.

For people with normal physiology most of these activities can be accomplished in comfort or at least with 'enjoyable' stress. Unfortunately, many people with lung disease have difficulty performing even normal daily activities without discomfort due to breathlessness. Such individuals complain of being 'short of breath' or 'unable to get their breath'. This difficulty in breathing is called dyspnoea and is frequently the reason for stopping exercise. Dyspnoea, like pain, is difficult to quantitate; however, it is an important symptom which commonly occurs in many respiratory diseases. In this chapter the physiology related to exercise and training will be described, and the types of respiratory problems that cause dyspnoea and limit exercise capacity will be discussed. The therapeutic interventions suitable for the management of such problems will be described.

EXERCISE PHYSIOLOGY

The three major body systems involved in exercise are the neuromuscular system, the cardiovascular system, and the respiratory system. Each system is driven by muscular power, whether skeletal, cardiac or respiratory. The ability of a person to exercise depends on the integrity of each of these systems. In this section, the relationship between the integrity of the respiratory system and exercise is highlighted.

Energy for muscular exercise is derived when adenosine triphosphate (ATP) is converted to adenosine diphosphate (ADP) and inorganic phosphate (Pi) by the action of the enzyme adenosine triphosphatase which is present in myosin within the muscle.

131

$$ATP \rightarrow ADP + Pi + ENERGY$$

There is a small amount of ATP present in the muscle which provides energy, by the above reaction, when exercise is initiated. However, for muscular contraction to continue, a larger supply of ATP must be available. Three different chemical reactions provide ATP depending on the type of exercise and its duration. Two of these reactions do not require oxygen and are only able to provide relatively small amounts of ATP. The third reaction requires oxygen and provides abundant ATP allowing exercise to continue for longer. A properly functioning respiratory system is vital for the provision of an adequate oxygen supply to the muscles so that this reaction can occur. In more detail, the three reactions that can provide ATP are:

1   At the beginning of exercise ATP can be reformed instantaneously from creatine phosphate (CP) stores within the muscle. This reaction is catalysed by the enzyme creatine phosphokinase (CPK).

$$CP + ADP \xrightarrow[CPK]{} C + ATP$$

The supply of CP is limited and CP stores are only adequate for about 9 sec of a 10-sec 100-metre run.

2   ATP can still be provided once the stores of CP are depleted. This involves the breakdown of glucose and glycogen in the following reaction:

$$glucose/glycogen + P_i + ADP \rightarrow H^+ + lactate + ATP$$
$$(H^+ = hydrogen\ ion)$$

This reaction does not require oxygen and is known as *anaerobic* (without air) *metabolism*. The energy output from anaerobic metabolism is relatively small, consequently the amount of exercise that can be performed under anaerobic conditions is limited. Anaerobic metabolism is usually required during exercise of high intensity and short duration.

3   ATP can be provided for exercise by utilizing oxygen (O_2) in a reaction with carbohydrates (such as glucose), fats or proteins (proteins are not readily used except in conditions of starvation).

$$Glucose/FFA + O_2 + P_i + ADP \rightarrow H_2O + CO_2 + ATP$$
$$(FFA = free\ fatty\ acids)$$

This is known as *aerobic metabolism*. It is a more efficient type of metabolism since glucose can supply 20 times more energy per mol, aerobically than anaerobically. Aerobic metabolism is the only type of metabolism that can provide energy for exercise of longer duration. The increased oxygen supply to the muscle required for aerobic exercise is provided by enhanced respiratory and cardiovascular responses. Any malfunction within the respiratory or cardiovascular systems may affect the supply of oxygen and reduce the capacity for prolonged exercise.

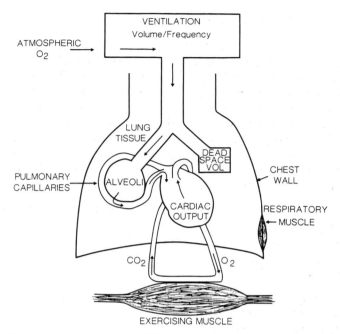

Figure 7.1   Diagrammatic representation of the movement of oxygen (O_2) from the atmosphere to the exercising muscle. CO_2 = carbon dioxide.

Figure 7.1 shows how the respiratory and cardiovascular systems provide oxygen to the muscles. Oxygen moves from the atmosphere into the lungs by the action of the respiratory muscles on the rib cage and abdomen. The respiratory muscles and rib cage act together as a 'bellows' which pumps air into and out of the lungs through the airways. The oxygen arrives at the alveoli where it transfers, by diffusion, into the pulmonary capillary bed. The heart pumps the blood carrying the oxygen to the working muscles. At the muscle level, oxygen diffuses into the muscle mitochondria, aided by enzymes.

The increased demand for oxygen required for exercise is met by an increase in both ventilation and cardiac output. During heavy exercise *pulmonary ventilation* per minute ($\dot{V}_E$) normally increases from a resting 6 litres per minute to 100, 150 or even 200 litres per minute in order to supply adequate oxygen to the working muscles and to remove carbon dioxide (CO_2). This is accomplished by increases in both tidal volume (V_t) and the frequency of breathing (f_b).

$$V_E = V_t \times f_b$$

At low to moderate workloads the increase in ventilation is mainly achieved by an increase in tidal volume. This continues until tidal volume reaches approximately 50% of vital capacity (VC). The increase in tidal volume is mainly in the direction of the inspiratory reserve volume. The

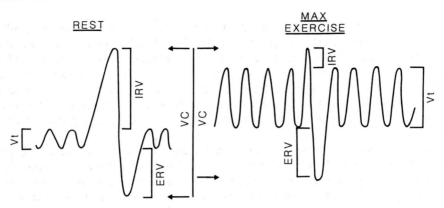

Figure 7.2   Changes in tidal volume (Vt) from rest to exercise. IRV = inspiratory reserve volume; ERV = expiratory reserve volume; VC = vital capacity.

expiratory reserve volume changes little (Figure 7.2). At high levels of exercise the increase in ventilation is a result of an increase in breathing frequency. The frequency of breathing ranges from a resting rate of 10–20 breaths per minute to a possible 40–50 breaths per minute in healthy subjects. This pattern of increasing ventilation first by increasing tidal volume and then by increasing frequency of breathing is so that a particular ventilation is achieved at optimal efficiency, that is, with the utilization of a minimum of energy by the respiratory muscles.[1] As circumstances change, an individual's pattern of breathing will alter in a bid to meet the ventilatory needs in the most energy efficient way. Although only 50% of the vital capacity is normally used during exercise, it can be seen from Figure 7.2 that the maximum tidal volume available is limited by the size of the vital capacity. This will become important in disease states where vital capacity is reduced.

The *cardiac output* (Q) increases from approximately 5 litres per minute at rest to 25 litres per minute during heavy work. This is accomplished by increases in both heart rate (HR) and stroke volume (SV).

$$Q = HR \times SV$$

The distribution of cardiac output alters markedly during exercise with an increased proportion being directed to the working skeletal muscles and to the skin. The purpose of this is to allow maximum supply of oxygen to the working muscles and to remove the metabolic heat produced by those muscles.

TRAINING

Endurance training (as opposed to strength training) modifies the responses of the respiratory and cardiovascular systems to exercise by improving the ability of the muscles to extract oxygen. Following training there is a substantial increase in the number and density of mitochondria and in the concentrations of the enzymes involved in oxidative metabolism in the trained muscles. Also the capillary density increases, providing greater blood supply to the muscle fibres. Skeletal muscle myoglobin increases, allowing improved diffusion of oxygen into the muscle. The principal consequence of these changes is greater extraction of oxygen by the trained muscles.

In the *respiratory system*, the improved oxygen extraction at the exercising muscle level results in a lower ventilatory requirement for exercise of moderate to high intensity. The ventilatory requirement at low intensity exercise is unchanged. The reason for this is that, at low levels of work, ventilation is driven by carbon dioxide production which is directly related to oxygen utilization. Pulmonary ventilation per litre of oxygen consumed does not therefore change greatly at this level of exercise after training. However, during heavier work, ventilation is not only stimulated by carbon dioxide production but also by the increase in blood lactate. The improved oxygen extraction at the muscle level means that blood lactate levels are lower at these work intensities following training. This reduces respiratory drive and consequently lowers pulmonary ventilation.[2] This is of benefit to patients with respiratory disease since the demands on the respiratory system will be less following training. Training can also increase the maximum oxygen uptake allowing for higher workloads to be achieved. This means that the level of oxygen uptake required to perform particular submaximal activities would be at a lower percentage of maximum oxygen uptake after training. This enables such activities to be carried out with more ease. For example, housework requires an oxygen uptake of approximately 0.9 litres per minute,[3] if this represents a lower percentage of maximum the person will feel less dyspnoea doing this activity than if this was at a higher relative level.

In the *cardiovascular system*, the improved oxygen extraction at the muscle level following training decreases the demand for blood flow at a given metabolic rate. This means that the cardiac output required at an equivalent pre-training workload is lower and the heart rate is reduced. This is of great benefit to patients with cardiac disease, since cardiac work is reduced and, as a consequence of the decreased heart rate, the diastolic period when the coronary vessels are best perfused, is increased (see Chapter 8).

In order to achieve the benefits of training, various exercise programmes have been devised. The programmes are designed so that the person undertakes a training load of sufficient intensity, duration and frequency to produce a training effect.[2,4] The optimal training stimulus will vary from one individual to another depending on the initial level of fitness, age, etc. For untrained people, a work intensity that requires an oxygen uptake of more than 50% of the person's maximum may be sufficient to produce a training effect.[2] Training at a higher intensity will achieve even better results[5] although this may be too stressful for many individuals with respiratory disorders. The duration and frequency component of the training stimulus can be varied according to individual needs and lifestyles. However, 20–30 minutes exercise five times per week will give the best results.[5]

To determine accurately that a person is working above 50% of his/her maximum oxygen uptake, a maximum exercise test is required. For this, the subject performs exercise on either a stationary bicycle or treadmill while changes in heart rate, ventilation, oxygen utilization and carbon dioxide production are recorded. The workload is increased every 1–2 minutes until the subject cannot exercise any further. From this test the maximum oxygen uptake can be calculated[3] and the heart rate achieved at 50% of maximum oxygen uptake, found. An exercise programme is then devised so that the person works slightly above this heart rate. If no such assessment is available, an elevation of the heart rate by about 60 beats per minute above resting level may be a suitable intensity. Another guide used is to exercise at a heart rate of 195 minus the person's age in years.[2] This should result in a submaximal level of exercise. In people with respiratory disease, it is applicable to base training intensity on heart rate in those individuals whose lung disease still allows them to exercise at moderately high heart rates. On the other hand, individuals with severe respiratory impairment may not achieve very high exercise heart rates as they stop exercise at relatively low work rates due to severe dyspnoea. In such people, the heart rate may not be a good guide for training intensity and programmes may need to be based on exercising at the level of ventilatory limitation. The rationale for this is that such individuals will habituate to the level of dyspnoea experienced during training and therefore be able to exercise for longer before dyspnoea limits their activity.[6]

The most effective exercises for achieving a training effect are those that involve a large muscle mass, for example, the legs.[4] Most training programmes for persons with respiratory disorders offer such activities as walking on the flat or up an incline on the treadmill,[7,8,9] stationary bicycling,[10,11] stair climbing.[12] These activities are appropriate as most are required as part of normal daily life so the biochemical changes brought about by such training will improve exercise tolerance for daily activities. A number of investigators have shown that some individuals with chronic airflow limitation who cannot exercise at intensities high enough to stimulate biochemical changes still show improvement in exercise tolerance following a training programme.[7,8,9,11,13] This ability to perform more exercise has been attributed to better economy of movement in the training activity,[14] increased tolerance to the sensation of dyspnoea[6,15] and increased confidence and motivation.[15]

Bicycle riding, although less likely to be performed by individuals in their daily lives, is useful as a training device as it supports the body weight enabling exercise to begin at a low level even in obese individuals. Bicycling also enables accurate determination of the work rate and allows for easy monitoring of the pulse rate as the upper body is steady. In some individuals with chronic airflow limitation, fixing the shoulder girdle by resting the arms on the handle-bars may enable them to achieve a greater work level by allowing improved function of the accessory muscles of breathing.[16] If bicycle training results in improved muscular efficiency in extracting oxygen, some of this improvement will be transferable to walking[14] as similar muscle masses are involved. However, as a proportion of the training effect in people with chronic airflow limitation is attributed to improved economy of movement in the training activity,[14] exercise programmes should mostly involve those activities that cause the individual most limitation.

For patients who are particularly limited and cannot perform the above exercise without great distress, single limb endurance exercise may be of benefit. Single limb bicycle exercise can be performed at a lower ventilation and does not, therefore, cause the same degree of dyspnoea as bilateral limb exercise. In normal subjects, single leg endurance training results in similar peripheral changes in the exercising muscle groups as seen in two-legged exercise.[17] However, in people whose exercise tolerance is severely limited the intensity of exercise may not be great enough to elicit such changes. The benefit of single limb exercise for these people may be improved economy of movement in the training task.

Arm exercise presents a special problem for individuals with severe ventilatory limitation. Often these individuals fix their shoulder girdle by resting their arms on a firm surface so that the accessory muscles of respiration can pull on the rib cage in an effort to shift more air in and out of the lungs. Activities involving the arms may mean loss of these arm–trunk muscles as muscles of respiration.[18] In addition, elevation of the arms, such as in combing the hair, decreases perfusion pressure to the arm muscles. With a reduced blood supply, lactate accumulates at a very low metabolic rate and may prevent further activity.[19] Specific arm muscle training could lead to reduced lactic acid production and better coordination of breathing movements during arm activity.[20] This would allow sustained dynamic exercise of the arms, such as shaving and hair combing, to be done in more comfort.

A training programme should be tailored to each individual bearing in mind specific needs. The results of training will vary from individual to individual depending on the extent of the training stimulus. This in turn is affected by motivation[15] and the degree to which the respiratory impairment limits the intensity of exercise performed.[13]

ANALYSIS OF RESPIRATORY PROBLEMS THAT LIMIT EXERCISE CAPACITY

The ability to supply oxygen to the working muscles can be affected by pathological processes within the respiratory system. The following processes result in inadequate ventilation or gas exchange which reduces the amount of oxygen available to the working muscles leading to a limited exercise capacity.

1   Airway narrowing causing *limitation to airflow* which occurs in obstructive lung diseases such as emphysema, chronic bronchitis, asthma, cystic fibrosis.
2   A *reduction in volume of the lung* due to abnormalities of the lung tissue which cause lung stiffness, as in pulmonary fibrosis; or abnormalities of the chest wall such as kyphoscoliosis following poliomyelitis.
3   A *reduction* in the ability to *transfer oxygen* from the lungs into the pulmonary capillary blood either because of mismatching of ventilation and perfusion, as in emphysema, or because of diffusion abnormalities, as in pulmonary fibrosis.
4   An increase in the *oxygen cost of breathing*.
5   *Respiratory muscle weakness or fatigue* which reduces the ability of the respiratory muscles to generate power.

In the following sections the above changes will be elaborated and the implications for therapeutic intervention will be discussed.

AIRFLOW LIMITATION

One of the most common causes of exercise limitation is chronic airflow limitation (CAL) which can occur in disorders such as chronic bronchitis,* emphysema,* and cystic fibrosis (CF). These disorders limit work capacity by reducing the available maximal expiratory flow rates. In normal individuals during exercise, ventilation increases due to increases in both tidal volume and frequency of breathing. The increases in breathing frequency naturally require an increase in inspiratory and expiratory flow rates in order to shift the larger volume of air in a shorter time. There is, however, a limit to the maximum flow rates that can be achieved in any individual. This can be measured by maximal inspiratory and expiratory flow–volume curves (see Figure 3.11). Normal sedentary individuals do not reach their maximal expiratory flow rates when performing moderate exercise.[21] In fact there is a significant reserve between the exercising flow rates and the maximal possible expiratory flow rates. For this reason, flow rate is not thought to be a limiting factor to exercise in normal untrained people. People with CAL have reduced flow rates throughout the range of lung volumes, from total lung capacity to residual volume, causing limitation to air flow. This is seen graphically in the concave maximal flow–volume curve (see Figure 3.12c). Once these individuals reach their maximum flow rates during exercise, ventilation cannot be increased any more to cope with any increase in workload. In this way, work capacity is limited by the limitation to airflow. In people with severe airflow limitation, expiratory flow may be at maximum levels even during tidal breathing at rest.

* The term chronic obstructive lung disease (COLD) has been used to describe people with chronic bronchitis and emphysema, however, CAL is now a more commonly used term.

Many individuals with CAL have been shown to breathe at a higher lung volume during exercise, that is, they hyperinflate which is shown by an increase in the volume of gas left in the lungs at end tidal expiration.[22] This hyperinflation is beneficial in slightly reducing airflow limitation by causing the airways to be more open. In this way, such individuals can achieve higher expiratory flow rates (Figure 7.3) and consequently higher levels of ventilation which allow better work performance. The negative aspect is that hyperinflation places the inspiratory muscles at a mechanical disadvantage and increases the elastic work of breathing.

As well as the fact that limitation to airflow causes a reduction in exercise capacity, many individuals with CAL have a lowered exercise capacity due to arterial oxygen desaturation. In this situation it is often difficult to determine whether it is the limitation to airflow or the arterial oxygen desaturation which is mainly responsible for the reduced exercise capacity. However, there is evidence that airflow limitation alone can cause exercise limitation in people with CAL. This is demonstrated in a subgroup of individuals with moderately reduced exercise tolerance due to CAL who do not desaturate during heavy exercise, indicating that gas exchange is adequate and that the limitation to exercise is due to impairment of respiratory mechanics, that is, inability to increase ventilation.[23]

The aim of intervention is to reduce the underlying airflow limitation as this will result in improved ventilation and consequently an improved exercise tolerance. Airflow limitation may be reduced by appropriate drug therapy such as bronchodilators which reduce spasm of the bronchial smooth muscle, steroids which decrease inflammation and oedema of the airways, and by the clearance of bronchial secretions. Each of these, if effective, increases the size of the lumen of the airway and, therefore, allows better airflow.

People with airflow limitation can also be encouraged to participate in exercise training programmes in order to benefit from the training effect of

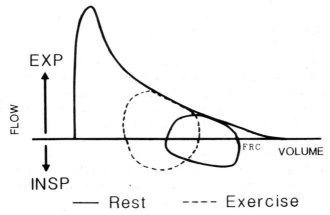

Figure 7.3 Tidal flow–volume loops at rest and during exercise in relation to the maximum expiratory flow–volume curve in a subject with airflow limitation.

an improved oxygen extraction at the muscle level. The improved oxygen extraction results in a decrease in ventilatory requirement at moderate workloads thus enabling the person to perform an equivalent pre-training level of activity with less dyspnoea following training. The improved oxygen extraction may also result in an increased aerobic capacity[24] which allows attainment of higher work intensities before ventilation becomes a limiting factor. However, the majority of individuals who present with CAL have such severe respiratory impairment that they cannot exercise at sufficient intensity for the changes at the muscle level associated with training to occur. In these individuals no metabolic training effect on skeletal muscle such as increased muscle oxidative enzymes has been shown.[13] Similarly, there has been shown to be no improvement in cardiac function following training.[7,13] Interestingly such people still benefit from training programmes. Several investigators[7,8,11,13] have found that physical training in people with CAL enables them to perform a given workload at a lower frequency of breathing, minute ventilation, carbon dioxide production and oxygen consumption. These changes have been attributed to increased tolerance to the sensation of dyspnoea, especially if individuals have trained near their ventilatory limit,[6] improved efficiency of movement,[14] and increased confidence and motivation.[15] The approach to exercise training in people with CAL would depend on the degree of ventilatory limitation to exercise and should be tailored to the individual according to the severity of the disease and the goals of treatment (see case examples A and C).

REDUCTION IN THE VOLUME OF THE LUNG OR CHEST WALL

Some disease processes result in a reduction in lung volumes and are known as restrictive lung diseases (see Figure 3.18). Since the maximum tidal volume is limited by the size of the vital capacity, the vital capacity determines the available 'working volume'. As ventilation = Vt × fb a reduction in maximum tidal volume can reduce the maximum possible ventilation and, in so doing, limit exercise capacity.

Lung volume can be reduced by decreased lung compliance as occurs in certain restrictive lung diseases such as pulmonary fibrosis and pneumoconiosis. The lung volumes are reduced because interstitial fibrosis has caused the lungs to become 'stiff'. This means that the compliance of the lung is decreased so that on inspiration a reduced number of lung units expand in response to a given transpleural pressure. A greater inspiratory effort is needed in order to achieve a required tidal volume. In this situation, the most efficient way to achieve the increased ventilation during exercise is by increasing the frequency of breathing in preference to increasing tidal volume. Lung volumes can also be reduced by chest wall defects such as occur in kyphoscoliosis and ankylosing spondylitis. The volume of the lung is reduced by stiffness and deformity of the external structures and this limits the ability to increase ventilation during exercise. These patients have normal lungs but their chest 'bellows' (muscles and rib cage) cannot develop the appropriate intrapleural pressures to expand the lungs sufficiently to achieve an adequate tidal volume for the required work. In both cases, these people breathe rapidly and shallowly during exercise. There is a limit to the degree to which the frequency of breathing can increase and still achieve an adequate exercise ventilation. This is due to the force–velocity characteristics of muscle. As the velocity of contraction increases, the force, that is, the pressure generated, decreases. The person cannot shift the same volume of air quickly so ventilation cannot increase after a certain frequency of breathing is reached. Thus exercise capacity for these people is limited by their inability to increase ventilation adequately.

Any intervention that can reduce the underlying cause of the lowered vital capacity will improve exercise capacity, for example, steroids to reduce pulmonary fibrosis, surgical correction of scoliosis. However, in most patients the limitation is fixed. Exercise programmes aimed at improving oxygen utilization at the muscle level, so that the demands on the ventilatory system are reduced at a given work intensity, will improve exercise tolerance. Such programmes may include exercise on a stationary bicycle or treadmill, walking or stair climbing.

ABNORMALITIES OF OXYGEN TRANSFER

Abnormalities of oxygen transfer can lead to hypoxaemia. This means that the working muscles will be undersupplied with oxygen with the consequent limitation to exercise. The most common forms of arterial hypoxaemia seen by the physiotherapist are those caused by ventilation/perfusion ($\dot{V}/\dot{Q}$) abnormalities and diffusion defects.

Mismatching of ventilation and perfusion means that some areas of the lung are well ventilated but not well perfused whereas others are well perfused but not well ventilated. This reduces gas exchange and if the mismatching is severe enough hypoxaemia occurs. $\dot{V}/\dot{Q}$ mismatching is responsible for most of the hypoxaemia seen in CAL. Individuals with $\dot{V}/\dot{Q}$ mismatching have a variable response to exercise in terms of the degree of oxygen desaturation. Some people with low initial oxygen saturations increase their saturation during exercise presumably by improving ventilation to already perfused areas of lung, whereas others desaturate even further due to inadequate ventilation indicated by increased end-tidal carbon-dioxide. Even when patients begin exercise with relatively good saturation, whether their oxygen saturation will increase or decrease during exercise cannot be predicted. However, results of lung function tests can help to predict which individuals will desaturate during exercise as it has been shown that desaturation is more likely to occur in those individuals with an FEV_1/VC ratio of less than 50%.[25] To know exactly which of the individuals with FEV_1/VC ratio of less than 50% will desaturate, a supervised exercise test with ear oximetry is required. On the basis of the test results it may be suggested that exercise be limited to a level which does not cause oxygen desaturation of more than 5% or a fall below an absolute saturation of 80%.[26] Exercise causing a fall in arterial saturation may contribute to the development of (or a worsening of) pulmonary hypertension, right ventricular hypertrophy and cor pulmonale. In addition, severe hypoxaemia induced by exercise may trigger ventricular arrhythmias.

Diffusion defects are another cause of hypoxaemia during exercise. Normally the oxygen levels throughout exercise remain stable. There is usually adequate transit time for the red blood cells to become fully saturated in the alveolar capillaries. This is the case even with the reduced transit time as a consequence of an increased cardiac output associated with exercise. However, when there is a diffusion abnormality, for example, in pulmonary fibrosis, even though there may be sufficient time for equilibrium across the alveolar membrane to occur at rest, on exercise, desaturation occurs progressively. Arterial hypoxaemia occurs despite exercise ventilation within the normal range and adequate perfusion. This is a result of the failure to achieve diffusion equilibrium because of the increased distance the oxygen has to travel due to the pulmonary fibrosis.

Individuals who become hypoxaemic during exercise and even those who are hypoxaemic at rest should not necessarily be excluded from exercise programmes. The degree of desaturation can be measured by ear oximetry during a standard progressive exercise test.[3] After adequate time for recovery the test should be repeated using supplemental oxygen to assess the effect on desaturation and work capacity. Carbon dioxide levels should also be documented to ensure that added oxygen does not have the detrimental effect of increasing carbon dioxide retention.

Supplemental oxygen usually results in an increased work capacity and a reduction in ventilation for an equivalent load performed with breathing air.[27] Individuals are, therefore, able to exercise at higher submaximal work rates without desaturation. This allows for a greater training stimulus. Improved efficiency of movement and increased tolerance to dyspnoea gained by such training may provide symptomatic relief during activities. These patients may require home oxygen to enable them to carry out daily activities. Every effort should be made to improve the oxygen transfer medically.

OXYGEN COST OF BREATHING

The respiratory muscles provide the driving force for ventilation. At rest, in normal people, the respiratory muscles only require 1–2% of the total oxygen uptake. Most of this oxygen consumption is used for the work required to overcome elastic recoil of the lungs and airways resistance. The size of the tidal volume determines the work to overcome elastic recoil, that is, expand the lungs on each breath. As tidal volume becomes greater, the work to overcome elastic recoil per minute increases. The flow rate, which is directly related to the frequency of breathing, determines the work to overcome airway resistance on each breath. As the rate becomes faster the 'resistive work' increases. Therefore, as ventilation (Vt × fb) increases with exercise so does the oxygen consumption of the respiratory muscles. During maximal exercise up to 10% of the total oxygen uptake may be required by the respiratory muscles in normal people.

When airways resistance is increased, as in asthma and CAL, more energy is needed to overcome resistance. Patients choose slow deep breathing to keep flow rates low and so avoid excessive resistive work. When these people exercise, ventilation increases requiring greater increases in resistive work. It has been estimated that the oxygen uptake of the respiratory system in patients with chronic obstructive pulmonary disease during moderate exercise is about 9 ml oxygen per litre of ventilation or 35–40% of total oxygen uptake.[28] The oxygen cost of breathing may become so great that the oxygen supply to other muscles is compromised and may limit further work. This is referred to as 'energy stealing', since the respiratory muscles 'steal' blood flow and energy potentially available for other working muscles.

Decreasing the work of breathing by reducing airway resistance with the use of appropriate drug therapy, for example, bronchodilators and steroids, will improve exercise performance. Endurance training that results in a decreased ventilation for a given workload will enable more work to be performed before the oxygen cost of breathing limits exercise.

RESPIRATORY MUSCLE WEAKNESS AND FATIGUE

Muscle weakness is defined as 'a condition in which the capacity of a rested muscle to generate force is impaired'. Muscle fatigue is defined as a 'condition in which there is a loss in the capacity for developing force and/or velocity of a muscle, resulting from muscle activity under load and which is reversible by rest'.[29] In terms of the respiratory muscles, fatigue means inability to continue generating a particular pleural pressure. Muscle fatigue, as opposed to central or neuromuscular transmission fatigue, occurs when the rate of energy consumption by a muscle is greater than the rate of energy supplied to the muscle by the blood. To continue contracting, the muscle draws on its energy stores. When these are depleted, energy supply is inadequate and the muscle fails as a force generator.

In normal, untrained subjects during moderate exercise there is no detectable respiratory muscle fatigue. However, patients with respiratory disease may show signs of respiratory muscle fatigue during exercise[30,31] and, in extremely severe cases, even at rest. This fatigue will limit a person's ability to maintain adequate ventilation for exercise. Indeed, it has been shown in normal subjects that reduced ventilatory muscle endurance induced by prior ventilatory work results in lower maximum exercise ventilation and consequently decreased exercise performance.[32]

There are many factors that influence the development of respiratory muscle fatigue:

1 Increased load on the respiratory muscles. This occurs in any disorders where airways resistance is increased, for example, CAL, acute asthma, and in other situations such as obesity. Respiratory muscles have to generate higher pleural pressures to achieve the same ventilation. The work of breathing is increased and may predispose the muscle to fatigue. This has been substantiated by studies in normal subjects which showed that inspiratory muscles became fatigued when the subjects breathed against a resistance.[33]

2 Weak respiratory muscles fatigue sooner than strong muscles performing the same task. Of particular interest to physiotherapists is the weakness of respiratory muscles due to deconditioning following prolonged assisted ventilation, or to paralysis, as in quadriplegia.

3 When a person is hyperinflated, as in CAL or acute asthma, the inspiratory muscles act in their shortened range. The maximum tension, and consequently the maximum inspiratory pressures that these muscles can develop for the same neural input and energy consumption is less at these higher lung volumes, that is, they will have to work harder to provide the same ventilation. This will make the respiratory muscles more vulnerable to fatigue. Research data[34] has shown that normal subjects breathing at higher lung volumes cannot sustain the same mouth pressures for a prolonged period of time.

4 If the oxygen content of the blood is reduced, the availability of ATP via aerobic metabolism is decreased. The oxygen content of the blood could be low in diseases that reduce diffusion, for example, diffuse pulmonary fibrosis, and those that reduce ventilation/perfusion, for example, CAL and cystic fibrosis with severe pulmonary disease. It has been shown that respiratory muscle fatigue occurs more rapidly in normal subjects at lowered inspired oxygen concentrations.[35]

5 A reduction in the availability of muscle fuels will lead to muscle fatigue. In human skeletal muscle glycogen depletion correlates significantly with muscle fatigue following exercise of prolonged duration.[36] This would suggest that prolonged work uses up available energy stores and predisposes the muscle to fatigue. Certainly it has been shown that inspiratory and expiratory muscle strength is reduced after marathon running.[37] In animal experiments (rats), there has been shown to be a marked reduction in the glycogen content of the respiratory muscles following five hours of swimming.[38]

6 The degree to which the muscles are trained will affect their ability to extract energy stores. It appears that the respiratory muscles respond to training in a similar manner to skeletal muscles.[39] Training improves the ability of the muscles to extract energy stores and so will help to make the muscles less vulnerable to fatigue.

There are a number of ways a physiotherapist may be able to assess whether or not respiratory muscle fatigue is present during or after exercise. When normal subjects breathe against fatiguing loads they alternate between predominantly using the diaphragm or the intercostal/accessory muscles to develop the necessary pressures.[40] When the diaphragm is used, the abdomen is displaced outwards and the rib cage expands. When the intercostal/accessory muscles are used the abdomen is displaced inwards as the rib cage expands (paradoxical breathing). This strategy of alternating the contribution of the various muscles may serve to protect the inspiratory muscles from exhaustion, that is, when one muscle group is working the other is resting. In quadriplegic individuals, the inability to alternate respiratory muscle groups has been suggested as a factor contributing to the development of inspiratory muscle fatigue at lower loads in these people than in normal subjects.[40] Observation of asynchronous or uncoordinated breathing should, therefore, alert the physiotherapist to the possibility of respiratory muscle fatigue.

Alternatively, if maximum mouth pressures are significantly reduced following exercise this could be an indication of muscle fatigue. It should be noted, however, that maximum mouth pressures could also be reduced if hyperinflation occurs during exercise, as this shortens the inspiratory muscles, preventing them from developing as much tension. If the patient is particularly breathless following exercise it may be difficult to get accurate mouth pressure readings. In this case, measurements should be taken regularly throughout the recovery period. If mouth pressures are consistently lower than before exercise, respiratory muscle fatigue is suspected.

A commonly used research tool for assessing respiratory muscle fatigue has been the frequency spectrum analysis of the electromyogram (EMG). The EMG signals are analysed to find out if the ratio of high frequency EMG signals to low frequency EMG signals decreases. It has been shown that a decrease in the frequency spectrum ratio of the EMG occurs before the diaphragm fatigues.[41]

Where respiratory muscle fatigue is thought to be the underlying factor limiting ventilation and consequently reducing exercise capacity, respiratory muscle training can be utilized. Leith and Bradley[39] were the first to show that ventilatory muscle strength and endurance could be increased by ventilatory muscle training in normal people. Since then a number of studies have demonstrated improvement of ventilatory muscle endurance following ventilatory muscle training programmes in patients with CAL,[31,42,43,44] CF[45] and quadriplegia.[40] Most studies concentrated on improving respiratory muscle endurance rather than strength, as an improved ability to breathe for prolonged periods against added loads (as occurs in increased airways resistance, or quadriplegia with a chest infection) is most beneficial to these patients.

There are a number of ways to provide a training load for the respiratory muscles:

1   Hyperpnoeic Loading

With hyperpnoeic loading the respiratory muscles contract very rapidly under a low external load.[39,45] The subject is required to maintain a target ventilation which corresponds to an appropriate training intensity which is usually 70–80% of maximum voluntary ventilation. To allow ventilation to continue without blowing off carbon dioxide, some mechanism must be incorporated into the circuit to maintain the carbon dioxide at normal levels. The apparatus required for this type of training normally needs careful monitoring and is cumbersome for home use.

2   Resistive Loading

With resistive loading the respiratory muscles contract slowly under a high external load.[31,40,42] The subject is required to reach a set pressure which corresponds to an appropriate training intensity which is usually 70–80% of maximum inspiratory mouth pressure. Resistive loading can be achieved by breathing through a fixed resistance at a known flow rate.

3   Intensive Upper Body Exercise

It has also been shown that intensive upper body exercise, such as swimming or canoeing, produces improvement in ventilatory muscle endurance in young people with cystic fibrosis and asthma.[45,46] For these people a sporting activity is often a more enjoyable way to train the respiratory muscles than a specific respiratory muscle training programme.

In order to improve the endurance of the respiratory muscles, the exercise prescription must not only consider the type of exercise but also the frequency, duration and intensity of exercise. The same principles apply as for training other skeletal muscles, that is, at least three times/week for at least 15 minutes (some people may need time to build up this duration and others will need a longer training stimulus), working towards an intensity of between 60–85% of their maximum capacity.

When assessing ventilatory muscle training programmes it is important to note that differences in results may occur due to differences in patient selection and variations in the intensity, duration and frequency of the programmes. This point is illustrated by comparing the results of three studies.[44,45,47]

Belman and Mittman[44] trained the respiratory muscles in patients with CAL by using specific ventilatory muscle training techniques and produced a 31% increase in ventilatory muscle endurance. In a similar group of subjects, Belman and Kendregan[47] attempted to train the respiratory muscles by using specific arm or leg exercise only. This resulted in no improvement in ventilatory muscle endurance. In both studies, the duration and frequency of the training were similar but there was a marked difference in the intensity of exercise in relation to the respiratory muscles. In the first study, ventilation during training was 79% of maximum voluntary ventilation (MVV) at the start of training, whereas, in the second study, ventilation was only approximately 50% of MVV. Thus the stimulus to produce a training effect in the respiratory muscles was less when only arm or leg exercise was used and could explain the fact that non-specific muscle training did not improve ventilatory muscle endurance. It is conceivable that patients with CAL cannot tolerate the high intensity of arm or leg exercise required to produce a training effect in the ventilatory muscles and that, in order to train the ventilatory muscles in these people, specific ventilatory muscle exercise is necessary.

In contrast, Keens and colleagues,[45] using a similar concept in ventilatory muscle training as Belman and Kendregan, showed that intensive upper body training (canoeing and swimming) improved the endurance of the ventilatory muscles of children with cystic fibrosis. These younger subjects with better pulmonary function were probably able to sustain higher levels of ventilation during exercise and presumably this level of ventilation was of an adequate intensity to produce a training effect on the ventilatory muscles.

These results have implications for programme design for individual patients. Where a patient is able to exercise at a sufficient intensity to achieve improvement in respiratory muscle endurance then it is desirable to do so for the added benefits of whole body exercise, that is, for training effects on the cardiovascular system. Some younger patients with cystic fibrosis or asthma may fall into this category. When patients cannot achieve such levels of exercise, such as many individuals with CAL, then specific ventilatory muscle training may be of benefit and should be incorporated into a general exercise training programme so that the person benefits from both types of training without undue stress. However, it should be noted that improved ventilatory muscle performance following training has only been shown to increase exercise performance in people whose exercise tolerance was initially limited by the development of respiratory muscle fatigue.[31]

In some instances of very severe respiratory impairment the respiratory muscles may show signs of fatigue at rest. In such cases exercise would only exacerbate the problem. For these people, resting the respiratory muscles may result in improved exercise performance. Rest for the respiratory muscles can be provided by the use of nasal intermittent positive-pressure ventilation (IPPV) at night.[48] In some cases rest may provide time for depleted glycogen stores to be replenished.

EXERCISE-INDUCED ASTHMA

Exercise-induced asthma (EIA) presents a specific form of respiratory limitation to exercise. Normally the airways respond to exercise with a transitory slight bronchodilatation which is probably due to a combination of increased sympathetic tone and a withdrawal of vagal tone. The airways of asthmatic individuals also respond to exercise with a mild bronchodilatation; however, at the cessation of 6–8 minutes of exercise bronchoconstriction occurs.[49] This bronchoconstriction is thought to be due to the increased rate of ventilation during exercise which causes a loss of water from the respiratory mucosa. The water loss increases the osmolarity of the respiratory tract and decreases the temperature resulting in a release of mediators from mast cells in the airway lumen and submucosa which cause contraction of bronchial smooth muscle and oedema of the bronchial vasculature.[49] The bronchoconstriction is associated with an increase in hyperinflation and a decrease in arterial oxygen tension.

EIA can be successfully managed in most cases with appropriate drug therapy. Administration of an aerosol beta adrenoceptor agonist or sodium cromoglycate (Intal) before exercise has been shown effectively to block EIA.[49]

Since an increased rate of ventilation appears to be the prime trigger of EIA, exercise training may be of benefit. Following training, a lower ventilatory rate is required for an equivalent pretraining workload. This lowered ventilation means that the trigger stimulus for EIA would be reduced. Conversely, a higher level of exercise would be required to raise the ventilatory rate to a point where asthma occurs. This is beneficial as the asthmatic individual can perform higher intensity exercise before inducing an attack of asthma. A further advantage of exercise training is the possibility of an increase in respiratory muscle endurance. Improved respiratory muscle endurance may be of benefit during a prolonged attack of asthma. EIA certainly should not act as a deterrent to exercise. There are numerous examples of elite athletes with well controlled EIA.

NUTRITIONAL STATUS AND EXERCISE

Poor nutritional status has been shown to affect exercise performance of patients with cystic fibrosis[50] and adds to the impairment of lung function in patients with emphysema.[51] Malnutrition leads initially to a loss of body fat and then to muscle wasting.[52] Loss of leg muscle mass would have a direct effect on exercise performance. Similarly, the respiratory muscles can become wasted when loss of lean tissue occurs.[53] This can result in impaired respiratory muscle strength[54] and reduced lung function[51] and thus cause further exercise limitation. Where this may be suspected the individual should be referred to the appropriate nutritional adviser.

PSYCHOLOGICAL LIMITATIONS TO EXERCISE

There can be many psychological reasons why people with lung disease will adopt a level of activity inconsistent with their physiological ability.[15,55,56] The most common is fear of dyspnoea. It is an unpleasant and frightening experience to be desperately short of breath. If this feeling is associated with certain activities then it is natural to avoid these activities. Other reasons are related to the social stereotyping of older people and of 'sick' people. Western society does not expect older people with chronic diseases to be active. Families tend to want to look after their loved ones and not see them stressed. Many people fear public swimming pools or exercising in the cold and wind as this may increase their risk of a respiratory infection.

These people may be offered the opportunity to exercise in the presence of trained health personnel while being monitored for oxygen saturation, heart rate and degree of dyspnoea. This provides reassurance and helps the person to overcome the fear of dyspnoea. At each activity level, dyspnoea should be managed carefully with intermittent rests and by using positions of comfort. Realistic short-term goals should be set which are rewarded with positive reinforcement. These goals should be consistent with the person's own social needs. For example, if a person needs to climb stairs to get into the house an appropriate stair-climbing goal should be set.

There are thought to be psychological benefits from regular exercise. Regular physical exercise has been associated with the sensation of 'feeling better'. The mechanisms underlying such psychological changes are still not clearly understood but may relate to the release of endorphins, the brain's naturally occurring opiate.

COMPLIANCE WITH EXERCISE PROGRAMMES

It is difficult to maintain compliance to an exercise programme whether dealing with young children, adolescents, adults or the elderly. Compliance may be enhanced by supervision, by monthly follow-up sessions, by use of patient diary cards, by group training programmes, and by adding variety to the programme by, for example, including sporting activities that the person enjoys. Offering convenient times and locations will also enhance compliance. There is a great need for incentives and motivational rewards to encourage subjects to continue the programmes.[57] Measurement of performance following a period of training may indicate improvement and, in so doing, increase compliance to the programme.

EVALUATION OF EXERCISE PROGRAMMES

The efficacy of exercise programmes needs to be evaluated in terms of whether the specific goals have been reached. For example, if a programme is aimed to increase the number of stairs climbed before dyspnoea prevents further activity, has the programme achieved this? Methods of evaluating programmes should be related to the type of exercise used in the programme and the facilities available. If there are no laboratory facilities, the 12-minute[58] or 6-minute[59] walk test designed for patients with CAL is a useful measure for walking programmes. The 6-minute walk test is now more commonly used as it takes less time and is less tiring for the patient and still gives comparable results. The patient walks as far as possible in 6 minutes and this can be compared to the distance walked in 6 minutes after a training programme. For fitter patients the distance covered in a 12-minute run can be compared before and after training.[60] If there are laboratory facilities available, more detailed measurements can be made of ventilation, heart rate, respiratory rate and work load achieved during an exercise test on a bicycle ergometer, treadmill or step test[2] before and after a training programme. In patients with chronic airflow limitation the measurements gained on a 12-minute walk test correlate well with work achieved on a bicycle ergometer test.[61] Subjective assessment of perceived exertion during exercise using the Borg Score[62] or similar dyspnoea scale could also be a useful guide to changes that occur with training. Depending on the results of such assessment and feedback from the patient, programmes can be altered accordingly.

While this chapter has dealt with some of the pulmonary limitations to exercise as discrete problems, there are in fact many situations where there is a more complex interaction of effects. A person may have a reduced vital capacity and a poor diffusing capacity or airflow limitation and respiratory muscle fatigue. Alternatively, there may be a pulmonary limitation to exercise and some other disability such as an amputation, coronary artery disease or peripheral vascular disease which may compound the limitation to exercise. The physiotherapist should consider the component problems in drawing up a plan of action. In this way individuals will be provided with exercise prescriptions that are suitable for their disorders and their needs.

CASE EXAMPLES

Case A

A 58-year-old man diagnosed with chronic airflow limitation (CAL) presents with breathlessness on exertion. His FEV_1 is 45% predicted, FVC 79% predicted and FEV_1/FVC is 49%. The flow–volume curve shows marked reduction in flow at all lung volumes, and his resting (or tidal breathing) expiratory flow equals his maximum expiratory flow on the maximum flow–volume curve. His body mass index (BMI) is 18 (normal range 20–25). He can walk 600 metres on the flat without stopping but can only climb one flight of stairs before he has to stop because of breathlessness. An exercise test with ear oximetry reveals that his oxygen saturation is 90% at rest dropping to 78% at maximum exercise. His maximum workload is 30 watts (= 180 kpm).

    The above information establishes that the patient has a greatly reduced exercise capacity due to:

1   Flow limitation as seen by the resting expiratory flow–volume curve equalling the maximum expiratory flow–volume curve. This indicates that flows cannot be increased significantly during exercise.
2   Hypoxaemia, as seen by the oxygen saturation falling to 78% during the maximum exercise test. This indicates ventilation/perfusion abnormality.

When planning an exercise programme, the specific needs of this individual should be taken into account, e.g. he lives in a terrace house with his bedroom upstairs; the shops are approximately 500 metres away.

The broad goals of intervention should include optimizing lung function to reduce flow limitation as much as possible, then gradually increasing exercise tolerance without causing undue hypoxaemia. These goals can be achieved by the following programme:

1   To optimize lung function bronchodilator therapy could be given followed by sputum removal, if either is applicable. Both of these, if effective, would help to increase the calibre of the airways and reduce flow limitation. Any improvement in flow should lead to an improvement in exercise capacity.
2   To improve exercise tolerance a hospital-based exercise programme which would enable the patient to breathe supplemental oxygen during exercise could be implemented. The aim would be to improve efficiency of movement and tolerance to dyspnoea to a level at which the patient can cope with stair climbing and walking to the shops with more ease.

The most appropriate exercise programme would be one that allows intermittent exercise as this is less stressful for someone with severe limitation than a programme that requires longer duration work. An intermittent or interval programme would include a 1-minute warm-up at 20% of maximum work capacity (W_{max}), 3 minutes at 60% W_{max}, 1-minute cool-down at 20% W_{max}, rest. Over the time of the training programme the number of repetitions and the workload of the above sequence is increased until the patient is doing six repetitions in one session at a workload of 75% W_{max} by the end of a 3-month programme. For this patient the choice of walking and stair climbing may be the most appropriate training activities. The programme should be carried out at least 3 times/week. A home programme should also be designed after discussion with the patient as to the local terrain and house layout. A stair climbing programme may involve climbing up and down two steps for 2 minutes, aiming at building up to five steps for 5 minutes. The walk programme would be based on the results of the 6- or 12-minute walk test.

The intensity of exercise needs to be carefully monitored to ensure that exercise does not cause distressing dsypnoea and exacerbate problems associated with hypoxaemia. The patient should be reassessed regularly to ensure that he is coping with the programme. In addition, as the patient has a low nutritional status (BMI = 18) a dietitian should be consulted as improvement in nutritional status may improve muscle function.

Case B

This 24-year-old man suffered an incomplete spinal cord lesion at C6–C7. His FEV_1 is 2.5 l (57% predicted), FVC is 3.0 l (54% predicted), FEV_1/FVC is 83%, maximum inspiratory mouth pressure (P_Imax) is 40% predicted. His general health is good, however he suffers repeated respiratory infections. He is able to propel himself in a wheelchair with effort.

The work of breathing in quadriplegic individuals is increased due to a reduction in lung compliance and increased rib cage stiffness which occurs with time following paralysis. This creates more work for the few functional inspiratory muscles. In addition, chest infections further increase the work of breathing.

Analysis of the lung function data establishes that this patient's muscle paralysis has resulted in a reduced VC, reduced P_Imax and that the work of breathing is increased due to lung and rib cage stiffness. Superimposed on this are the repeated chest infections which further compromise lung function and increase the load on the already weak respiratory muscles (P_Imax 40% predicted). In addition, without intercostal muscles actively stabilizing the rib cage there may be inefficiency of the functioning muscles. The patient may, therefore, be at risk of respiratory muscle fatigue and may benefit from respiratory muscle training. His ability to propel himself in a wheelchair is dependent on a few arm and shoulder girdle muscles. It would be valuable to strengthen these muscles and to improve their capacity for endurance exercise.

Broad goals of intervention should include: clearing the chest during a respiratory infection; training the respiratory muscles to optimum function; training the skeletal muscles to enhance the ability to propel the wheelchair.

To achieve these goals a treatment programme for this patient could include appropriate techniques for sputum removal (see Chapter 6). When the patient has recovered sufficiently from the acute chest infection, a respiratory muscle training programme using inspiratory resistances could be commenced. The training should be carried out in two 15-minute sessions each day, 6 days a week. The inspiratory resistance to be used is gauged by getting the patient to breathe through different degrees of inspiratory resistance and finding the maximum level that can be sustained for 15 minutes. Training is then commenced using this resistance. After 8 weeks the resistance should be reassessed and, if training has occurred, a new level of inspiratory resistance is determined which is then used for further training. The programme should also include arm and shoulder girdle strengthening exercises as well as a programme for increasing the patient's capacity for endurance exercise. Such a programme would entail propelling the wheelchair a certain distance in a given time each day. Gradually the distance covered in the same time would be increased.

Case C

A 19-year-old man with cystic fibrosis was referred to physiotherapy for an exercise programme. His FEV_1 is 67% predicted, FVC is 86% predicted, FEV_1/FVC is 72%, BMI is 21 (normal range 20–25). On a bicycle ergometer test with ear oximetry to maximum work capacity he achieved 68% of his predicted Wmax. The oxygen saturation at rest was 96% which fell to 91% at maximum exercise. His ventilation at maximum exercise in relation to his maximum voluntary ventilation ($V_E$max/MVV) was 75%. His sputum production was approximately 80 ml in a 24-hour period.

There are a number of factors that may be contributing to the patient's reduced exercise capacity. First, some airflow limitation is evident from the FEV_1/FVC ratio being less than 80%. Another factor contributing to airflow limitation is sputum in the airways. Secondly, oxygen desaturation from 96% to 91% indicates some ventilation/perfusion abnormality; however, the degree of the desaturation is minor and would not limit exercise. Thirdly, the ventilation at maximum exercise in relation to the maximum ventilation possible ($V_E$max/MVV) was high (75%). Normal untrained individuals only require 60–70% of their MVV at maximum work. This requirement for a higher relative ventilation may contribute to exercise limitation if exercise is prolonged because ventilatory muscle fatigue may become a factor if high levels of ventilation need to be maintained. Although a combination of factors has contributed to his reduced work capacity no one factor alone is particularly severe.

This patient is likely to benefit from an exercise training programme for a number of reasons. First, an exercise programme would help to maintain cardiorespiratory fitness as the disease progresses. In fact an improvement in cardiorespiratory fitness should be expected as this patient is still able to exercise to a considerable extent. Secondly, appropriate exercise training, i.e., upper body activities, may have a flow-over effect resulting in training of the respiratory muscles. This would be of benefit at times of added loads on the respiratory muscles such as might occur during a chest infection. Thirdly, exercise has been shown to aid sputum removal[63,64] which may mean the patient could reduce the time spent in postural drainage and physiotherapy. Fourthly, if the patient became involved in a team sport he would reap the psychological benefits of exercise, i.e., improved self-esteem plus the support gained from a group activity.

Planning the exercise programme should take into consideration the age of the person and any occupational or recreational needs he has. This person is a law student with a busy lecture timetable. He enjoys team sports but has not previously been on any formal exercise programme. To enhance compliance to an exercise regime it is important to capture the person's interest. With these younger individuals it is often better to interest them in a sporting activity as well as using a basic exercise programme.

The specific goals of treatment would be to optimize lung function before exercise and gradually to increase tolerance and enhance sputum removal with an exercise programme.

The programme for this person would include:

1 A bronchodilator, if applicable, and selected sputum removal techniques (see Chapter 6) to optimize lung function.
2 A walk/jog exercise programme which increases the heart rate to a level that he achieved at 50% of his W_{max} for 10 minutes of a 20-minute exercise period. The duration and intensity of exercise at this level should gradually be extended. There should be a 'warm-up' period to this level of exercise and a 'cool-down' at the end of each session. The exercise should be undertaken at least 3 times/week. Indoor cricket or tip football could be substituted for the walk/jog programme once or twice a week to add variety and provide the benefits of team involvement.

As this person is likely to be exercising without supervision, regular monthly contact should be maintained to enhance compliance to the programme. He may be encouraged to keep a diary which notes how often he exercises, any problems with exercise, and any improvement of symptoms with exercise, as this may provide a further impetus to continuing the programme. After six months his exercise tolerance should be re-evaluated with a maximum exercise test.

Although this patient's weight/height index is within the normal range (BMI = 21), decreased nutrition is often a problem for patients with cystic fibrosis due to the pancreatic involvement. Nutritional status should be checked regularly, therefore, and any problems referred to a dietitian, as adequate nutrition is important in maintaining ability to exercise.

REFERENCES

1. Milic-Emili G., Petit J.M. (1960). Mechanical efficiency of breathing. *J. Appl. Physiol.*, **15**, 359.
2. Astrand P-O., Rodahl K. (1986). Physical training. In *Textbook of Work Physiology*. New York: McGraw-Hill, pp. 412–485.
3. Jones N.L., Campbell E.J., Edwards R.T.H., *et al.* (1982). *Clinical Exercise Testing*, 2nd edn. Philadelphia: W.B. Saunders.
4. American College of Sports Medicine Position Statement (1978). The recommended quantity and quality of exercise for developing and maintaining fitness in healthy adults. *Med. Sci. Sports.*, **10** (3), vii.
5. Shephard R. (1968). Intensity, duration and frequency of exercise as determinants of the response to a training regime. *Int. Z. Physiol.*, **26**, 272.
6. Carter R., Nicotra B., Clark L., *et al.* (1988). Exercise conditioning in the rehabilitation of patients with chronic obstructive pulmonary disease. *Arch. Phys. Med. Rehabil.*, **69**, 118.
7. Chester E.H., Belman M.J., Bahler R.C., *et al.* (1977). Multidisciplinary treatment of chronic pulmonary insufficiency. 3. The effect of physical training on cardiopulmonary performance in patients with chronic obstructive pulmonary disease. *Chest*, **72**, 695.

8. Pierce A.K., Taylor H.F., Archer R.K., *et al.* (1964). Responses to exercise training in patients with emphysema. *Arch. Intern. Med.*, **113**, 28.

9. Nicholas J.J., Gilbert R., Gabe R., *et al.* (1970). Evaluation of an exercise therapy program for patients with chronic obstructive pulmonary disease. *Am. Rev. Respir. Dis.*, **102**, 390.

10. Alison J.A., Samios R., Anderson S.D. (1981). Evaluation of exercise training in patients with chronic airway obstruction. *Phys. Ther.*, **61**, 1273.

11. Vyas M.N., Banister E.W., Morton J.W., *et al.* (1971). Response to exercise in patients with chronic airway obstruction. 1. Effects of training. *Am. Rev. Respir. Dis.*, **103**, 390.

12. McGavin C.R., Gupta S.P., Lloyd E.L., *et al.* (1977). Physical rehabilitation for chronic bronchitis: results of a controlled trial of exercise at home. *Thorax*, **32**, 307.

13. Belman M.J., Kendregan B.A. (1981). Exercise training fails to increase skeletal muscle enzymes in patients with chronic pulmonary disease. *Am. Rev. Respir. Dis.*, **123**, 256.

14. Paez P.N., Phillipson E.A., Manangkay M., *et al.* (1967). The physiologic basis of training patients with emphysema. *Am. Rev. Respir. Dis.*, **95**, 944.

15. Argle D.P., Baum G.L., Chester E.H., *et al.* (1973). Multidiscipline treatment of chronic pulmonary insufficiency. 1. Psychological aspects of rehabilitation. *Psychosom. Med.*, **35**, 41.

16. Banzett R.B., Topulos G.P., Leith D.E., *et al.* (1988). Bracing the arms increases the capacity for sustained hyperpnea. *Am. Rev. Respir. Dis.*, **138**, 106.

17. Saltin B., Nazar K., Costill D.L., *et al.* (1976). The nature of the training response; peripheral and central adaptations to one-legged exercise. *Acta Physiol. Scand.*, **96**, 289.

18. Criner G.J., Celli B.R. (1988). Effect of unsupported arm exercise on ventilatory muscle recruitment in patients with severe chronic airflow obstruction. *Am. Rev. Respir. Dis.*, **138**, 856.

19. Bevegard S., Freyschuss U., Strandell T. (1966). Circulatory adaptation to arm and leg exercise in supine and sitting position. *J. Appl. Physiol.*, **21**, 37.

20. Casaburi R., Wasserman K. (1986). Exercise training in pulmonary rehabilitation. *N. Engl. J. Med.*, **314**, 1509.

21. Stubbing D.G., Pengelly L.D., Morse J.L.C., *et al.* (1980). Pulmonary mechanics during exercise in normal males. *J. Appl. Physiol.: Respirat. Environ. Exercise Physiol.*, **49**(3), 506.

22. Dodd D.S., Brancatisano T., Engel L.A. (1984). Chest wall mechanics during exercise in patients with severe chronic air-flow obstruction. *Am. Rev. Respir. Dis.*, **129**, 33.

23. Grimby G., Stiksa J. (1970). Flow-volume curves and breathing patterns during exercise in patients with obstructive lung disease. *Scand. J. Clin. Lab. Invest.*, **25**, 303.

24. Casaburi R., Patessio A., Ioli F., *et al.* (1991). Reductions in exercise lactic acidosis and ventilation as a result of exercise training in patients with obstructive lung disease. *Am. Rev. Respir. Dis.*, **143**, 9.

25. Henke K.G., Orenstein D.M. (1984). Oxygen saturation during exercise in cystic fibrosis. *Am. Rev. Respir. Dis.*, **129**, 708.

26. Cropp G.J., Pullano T.P., Cerny F.J., *et al.* (1982). Exercise tolerance and cardiorespiratory adjustments at peak work capacity in cystic fibrosis. *Am. Rev. Respir. Dis.*, **126**, 211.

27. Pierce A.K., Paez P.N., Miller W.F. (1965). Exercise training with the aid of portable oxygen supply in patients with emphysema. *Am. Rev. Respir. Dis.*, **91**, 653.

28. Levison H., Cherniack R.M. (1968). Ventilatory cost of exercise in chronic obstructive pulmonary disease. *J. Appl. Physiol.*, **25**, 21.

29. NHLBI Workshop Summary (1990). Respiratory muscle fatigue. *Am. Rev. Respir. Dis.*, **142**, 474.

30. Grassino A., Gross D., Macklem P.T., *et al.* (1976). Inspiratory muscle fatigue as a factor limiting exercise. *Bull. Europ. Physiopath. Resp.*, **15**, 105.

31. Pardy R.L., Rivington R.N., Despas P.J., *et al.* (1981). The effects of inspiratory muscle training on exercise performance in chronic airflow limitation. *Am. Rev. Respir. Dis.* **123**, 426.

32. Martin B., Heintzelman M., Chen H-I. (1982). Exercise performance after ventilatory work. *J. Appl. Physiol.: Respirat. Environ. Exercise Physiol.*, **52**, 1581.

33. Roussos C.S., Macklem P.T. (1977). Diaphragmatic fatigue in man. *J. Appl. Physiol.: Respirat. Environ. Exercise Physiol.*, **43**, 189.

34. Roussos C.S., Fixley M.S., Gross D., *et al.* (1976). Respiratory muscle fatigue in man at FRC and higher lung volumes. *Physiologist*, **19**, 345.

35. Jardim J., Farkas G., Prefaut G., *et al.* (1981). The failing inspiratory muscles under normoxic and hypoxic conditions. *Am. Rev. Respir. Dis.*, **124**, 274.

36. Bergstrom J., Hultman E. (1972). Nutrition for maximal sports performance. *JAMA*, **221**, 999.

37. Loke J., Mahler D.A., Virgulto J.A. (1982). Respiratory muscle fatigue after marathon running. *J. Appl. Physiol.: Respirat. Environ. Exercise Physiol.*, **52**, 821.

38. Gorski J., Namoit A., Giedrojc J. (1978). Effect of exercise on metabolism of glycogen and triglycerides in the respiratory muscles. *Pfluegers Arch.*, **377**, 251.

39. Leith D.E., Bradley M. (1976). Ventilatory muscle strength and endurance training. *J. Appl. Physiol.*, **41**, 508.

40. Gross D., Ladd H.W., Riley E.J., *et al.* (1980). The effect of training on strength and endurance of the diaphragm in quadriplegia. *Am. J. Med.*, **68**, 27.

41. Gross D., Grassino A., Ross W.R.D., *et al.* (1979). Electromyogram pattern of diaphragmatic fatigue. *J. Appl. Physiol.: Respirat. Environ. Exercise Physiol.*, **46**, 1.

42. Sonne L.J., Davis J.A. (1982). Increased exercise performance in patients with severe COPD following inspiratory resistive training. *Chest*, **81**, 436.

43. Levine S., Weiser P., Gillen J. (1986). Evaluation of a ventilatory muscle endurance training program in the rehabilitation of patients with chronic obstructive pulmonary disease. *Am. Rev. Respir. Dis.*, **133**, 400.

44. Belman M.J., Mittman C. (1980). Ventilatory muscle training improves exercise capacity in chronic obstructive pulmonary disease patients. *Am. Rev. Respir. Dis.*, **121**, 273.

45. Keens T.G., Krastins I.R.B., Wannamaker E.M., *et al.* (1977). Ventilatory muscle endurance training in normal subjects and patients with cystic fibrosis. *Am. Rev. Respir. Dis.*, **116**, 853.

46. Schnall R., Ford P., Gillam I., *et al.* (1982). Swimming and dry land exercises in children with asthma. *Aust. Paediatr. J.*, **18**, 23.

47. Belman M.J., Kedregan B.A. (1982). Physical training fails to improve ventilatory muscle endurance in patients with chronic obstructive pulmonary disease. *Chest*, **81**, 440.

48. Ellis E.R., Bye P.T.B., Bruderer J.W., *et al.* (1987). Treatment of respiratory failure during sleep in patients with neuromuscular disease. *Am. Rev. Respir. Dis.*, **135**, 148.

49. Anderson S.D. (1988). Exercise-induced asthma. In *Allergy Principles and Practice*, 3rd edn (Middleton E., ed.). Washington: C.V. Mosby, pp. 1156–1175.

50. Marcotte J.E., Canny G.J., Grisdale R., *et al.* (1986). Effects of nutritional status on exercise performance in advanced cystic fibrosis. *Chest*, **90**, 375.

51. Openbrier D.R., Irwin M.M., Rogers R.M., *et al.* (1983). Nutritional status and

lung function in patients with emphysema and chronic bronchitis. *Chest*, **83**, 17.
52. Coates A.L., Boyce P., Muller D., *et al.* (1980). The role of nutritional status, airway obstruction, hypoxia, and abnormalities in serum lipid composition in limiting exercise tolerance in children with cystic fibrosis. *Acta Paediatr. Scand.*, **69**, 353.
53. Arora N.S., Rochester D.F. (1982). Effect of body weight and muscularity on human diaphragm muscle mass, thickness, and area. *J. Appl. Physiol.: Respirat. Environ. Exercise Physiol.*, **52**, 64.
54. Szeinberg A., England S., Mindorff C., *et al.* (1985). Maximal inspiratory and expiratory pressures are reduced in hyperinflated, malnourished, young adult male patients with cystic fibrosis. *Am. Rev. Respir. Dis.*, **132**, 766.
55. Argle D.P., Baum G.L. (1977). Physiological aspects of chronic obstructive pulmonary disease. *Med. Clin. North Am.*, **61**, 749.
56. Sandhu H.S. (1986). Psychosocial issues in chronic obstructive pulmonary disease. *Clinics in Chest Medicine*, **7**, 629.
57. Holzer F.J., Schnall R., Landau L.I. (1984). The effect of a home exercise programme in children with cystic fibrosis and asthma. *Aust. Paediatr. J.*, **20**, 297.
58. McGavin C.R., Gupta S.P., McHardy G.J.R. (1976). Twelve-minute walking test for assessing disability in chronic bronchitis. *Br. Med. J.*, **1**, 822.
59. Butland R.J.A., Pang J.A., Gross E.R., *et al.* (1981). Two, six and twelve-minute walks compared. *Thorax*, **36**, 225.
60. Cooper K.H. (1970). *The New Aerobics*. New York: Bantam Books Inc., pp. 29–30.
61. Alison J.A., Anderson S.D. (1981). Comparison of two methods of assessing physical performance in patients with chronic airway obstruction. *Phys. Ther.*, **61**, 1278.
62. Borg G. (1970). Perceived exertion as an indication of somatic stress. *Scand. J. Rehabil. Med.*, 92.
63. Zach M.S., Purrer B., Oberwaldner B. (1981). Effects of swimming on forced expiration and sputum clearance in cystic fibrosis. *Lancet*, **2**, 1201.
64. Zach M., Oberwaldner B., Hausler F. (1982). Cystic fibrosis: physical exercise versus chest physiotherapy. *Arch. Dis. Child.*, **57**, 587.

FURTHER READING

Bye P.T.P., Farkas G.A., Roussos CH. (1983). Respiratory factors limiting exercise. *Annu. Rev. Physiol.*, **45**, 439.
Derenne J-Ph., Macklem P.T., Roussos CH. (1978). The respiratory muscles: mechanics, control, and pathophysiology. *Am. Rev. Respir. Dis.*, **118**, 119–113 (part 1), 373–390 (part 2), 581–601 (part 3).
Wasserman K., Whipp B.J. (1975). Exercise physiology in health and disease. *Am. Rev. Respir. Dis.*, **112**, 219.

Chapter 8

Exercise Rehabilitation in Cardiac Disease

KATHY HENDERSON

INTRODUCTION

Medical and surgical techniques available for the management of cardiac patients have improved immeasurably in recent years. These improvements have undoubtedly added years to the lives of many cardiac patients. Physiotherapy intervention aimed at optimizing function may help to add quality of life by increasing capacity for work, recreation and general physical activity thereby helping to normalize lifestyle. There are few cardiac patients who would not benefit from an appropriate exercise intervention. It is critical, however, that the exercise is judiciously selected and the patients have a realistic understanding of its potential benefits and their own limitations.

Physiotherapy intervention for the individual with cardiac problems may range from bed exercises and chest care aimed at maintaining function in the bedridden patient, from education and counselling regarding lifestyle modification, to vigorous exercise conditioning suitable for selected patients in the later stages of rehabilitation. Also important are the specific chest care techniques used in the early postoperative treatment of patients who have undergone cardiac surgery.

Physiological studies have demonstrated the deconditioning effects likely to result from bedrest. Healthy young men put to bed for three weeks had a 20–25% decrease in their functional capacity.[1] Other deleterious effects may include postural hypotension, venous thrombosis, decreased pulmonary function and negative nitrogen and calcium balance.[2,3] More recent studies have indicated that many of these effects may be minimized simply by exposure to gravity.[4] This means that patients should sit on the edge of the bed or at the bedside as soon as their condition is stable enough to tolerate this.

Most patients benefit from increased understanding of coronary risk factors and also welcome advice regarding strategies for their management or modification. Risk factors may be defined as those habits and bodily characteristics associated with an increased chance of developing coronary heart disease. They should not be considered as causes of heart disease. Some patients with arteriopathy do not have any risk factors and others with multiple risk factors never develop heart disease. Risk factors include smoking, hypertension, hyperlipidaemia, diabetes mellitus, sedentary habits and stressful lifestyles.

The cardiac patients usually considered to require rehabilitation are those with coronary heart disease. Both patients who have recently suffered a myocardial infarction and those following coronary artery bypass surgery would be included in this group although the management will vary slightly. Other patients who may also benefit from rehabilitation include those with valvular heart disease, valve replacement surgery, cardiomyopathy, Barlow's syndrome and some rhythm disturbances. The principles of treatment are very similar for all these groups of patients. When planning a rehabilitation programme for any patient, the pathology and its effects on the haemodynamics should always be considered. Frequently the onset of signs and symptoms of heart disease is sudden and patients have no prior suspicion they have any health problems. They are usually not prepared either physically or psychologically for its implications and outcomes.

CARDIAC REHABILITATION

Comprehensive cardiac rehabilitation is a multifaceted process and professionals from many backgrounds may have contributions to make to the overall process. Depending on the facilities and staff available, team members participating in cardiac rehabilitation may vary widely. The physiotherapist has an ideal educational background to be a valuable team member and, circumstances permitting, should always seek to make some contribution to the rehabilitation process. Other team members who may be involved include medical and nursing staff, dietitian, occupational therapist, social worker and pharmacist.[5]

According to the World Health Organization and experts of the International Society of Cardiology:

> ... The rehabilitation of cardiac patients can be defined as the sum of activities required to ensure them the best possible physical, mental and social conditions, so that they may by their own efforts, regain as normal as possible a place in the community and lead an active productive life.[6]

An important component of this definition is that 'by their own means' the patients return to an active, productive lifestyle. Rehabilitation staff cannot make lifestyle changes for their patients. The patients must firstly be convinced of the potential benefits of such modifications and want to introduce them and secondly, be helped to plan and institute the change in lifestyle in a safe and practical manner. Some patients may decide they do not want to change their habits and lifestyle and this is their choice, however unwise others may believe them to be.

TABLE 8.1

Complications following myocardial infarction or cardiac surgery requiring special consideration or postponement of early cardiac rehabilitation

CRITERIA FOR CLASSIFICATION OF COMPLICATED MYOCARDIAL INFARCTION

Continued cardiac ischaemia (pain, late enzyme rise)
Left ventricular failure (congestive heart failure, new murmurs, X-ray changes)
Shock (blood pressure drop, pallor, oliguria)
Important cardiac arrhythmias
Conduction disturbances
Severe pleurisy or pericarditis
Complicating illnesses

SPECIAL CONSIDERATIONS FOR PATIENTS FOLLOWING CARDIAC SURGERY

Febrile (temperature greater than 102°F)
Sinus tachycardia (greater than 120 beats per minute at rest)
Symptomatic anaemia (haematocrit less than 30%)
Wound infection
Unstable sternum

The modern approach to cardiac rehabilitation revolves around the early mobilization of patients who do not have complications. This early ambulation is based on controlled clinical studies which did not find a greater incidence of death or other complications in patients mobilized early compared to patients who remain on bed rest longer.[3] When combined with optimal medical management and appropriate education, early mobilization helps people quickly to return to a healthy, active and productive lifestyle. Early mobilization is only suitable for those who do not have complications. Patients with complications of myocardial infarction (MI) or cardiac surgery, such as those listed in Table 8.1, should have mobilization delayed until complications are resolved.

Traditionally cardiac rehabilitation is divided into three phases with essential medical, educational and exercise components being applied during each phase. Each patient's rate of progression through these phases will vary depending on the nature and severity of illness, complications and rate of recovery. Those who have complications requiring prolonged hospitalization or further investigations may have to have progress through the phases delayed until their condition has stabilized.

Phase I is the acute in-hospital phase. It is usually 7–14 days in duration. The goals of rehabilitation during this phase are maintenance of functional capacity, development of patient confidence, minimization of anxiety and depression, and maximization of the chance of early discharge.

Medical objectives during Phase I include stabilizing the patient, controlling pain and arrhythmias as well as limiting the extent of myocardial damage. The educational objectives are initially to settle the patient into the coronary care unit and explain the pathology. During the latter part of hospitalization, risk factors are identified and individuals helped to plan appropriate lifestyle modifications. The exercise component during this stage is concerned with early mobilization aiming to minimize the deconditioning effects of prolonged bed rest whilst reassuring the patient that it will be possible to resume physical activity following this cardiac event.

During Phase I the rate of progression of people who have had a myocardial infarction is slightly slower than for those who have had coronary artery bypass grafts. Mobilization of surgical patients usually starts earlier and intensity and duration of ambulation are more accelerated. Activities commonly utilized in inpatient programmes include walking, upper limb exercises and stair climbing. Useful clinical indicators of appropriate exercise intensity in this phase include patient comfort, lack of dyspnoea, palpitations or dizziness and increase in pulse of less than twenty beats per minute. It is important to emphasize upper limb exercises for surgical patients in order to minimize the adhesions, muscle shortening and atrophy which may occur secondary to the sternotomy.[7] If left unchecked these can result in persistent poor posture or inability to regain preoperative strength.

Most cardiac units utilize a day-to-day activity plan as the basis for mobilization and education of all patients. These types of plans outline progressive stages of mobilization and education. Rate of progression through the programme can be varied from patient to patient and guided by the physician in charge. Mobilization achievements and education given can be recorded on a chart. This is particularly helpful when several staff members may be contributing to the patient's rehabilitation, saving confusion or unnecessary duplication. Examples of suitable charts can be found in Metier, Pollock and Graves[8] and Wenger.[2]

Phase II is the early convalescent phase (8–12 weeks in duration) and commences when the patient is discharged from hospital. During this phase myocardial and/or postoperative healing is taking place. By 6–8 weeks following the event both surgical and myocardial infarction patients are becoming ready to adopt a normal lifestyle as myocardial scar formation has taken place and the sternum is healed following surgery.

Medical objectives during this time include maintaining medical stability, adjusting medications and undertaking ongoing investigations such as exercise testing, echocardiography or angiography as necessary. The educational goals are to reinforce the need for lifestyle modification providing encouragement and support as necessary. Exercise during this time is gradually increasing in frequency and intensity with a corresponding increase in activities of daily living.

A well-balanced Phase II programme aims to have patients back to all of the activities of daily living consistent with a healthy lifestyle by the time healing is complete and a tough scar has formed. It is important to consider the patient's previous lifestyle and physical limitations. It is unrealistic to expect a patient to be more active after an MI than before if there are other factors limiting exercise capacity. Often, however, at this stage patients feel fitter than they did just prior to their cardiac event.

Phase III is the long-term reconditioning phase which will, if necessary, prepare the patient for return to heavy work and previous active recreation. Medical management continues to maintain cardiovascular stability, adjusting or instituting medications as necessary. Education continues to support lifestyle modification and the dose of exercise is increased to have a cardiovascular conditioning effect.

Exercise is considered by many[2,9] to be the cornerstone of cardiac rehabilitation, especially in the out-patient Phases II and III. The exercise component of these phases may be conducted as either a supervised programme where patients attend a facility on a regular basis to exercise under supervision or as a home programme in which the exercise is prescribed in a similar manner but is unsupervised and undertaken by the patients on their own. Each of these approaches has relative merits.[10] Supervised programmes provide additional support for patients who are not confident in their ability to exercise. Such groups are also a useful avenue for evaluating patients who may be having difficulty with resuming normal activity. The commitment to exercising with a group helps maintain motivation for many patients who would otherwise comply poorly with their exercise regime. Supervised programmes, however, are more expensive to run and are more time consuming for patients than exercising unsupervised at home. Some patients can become dependent on the group support and be unable to continue their exercise unsupervised following discharge from the group.

EXERCISE PRESCRIPTION

Exercise should be prescribed with the same precision as any medication. It is not adequate to tell a patient to 'do a bit more' or 'become more active'. The patient should be encouraged to have a balanced outlook and realistic expectations. The aim is not to produce 'exercise junkies' or to set standards so high they seem unattainable for the patient, who may then become discouraged and non-compliant.

The principles employed in prescribing exercise for the cardiac patient are the same as those for the healthy adult. The purpose of the prescription is to provide a level of exercise which will be safe while stimulating an improvement in functional capacity and an enhanced feeling of well-being. It should be based on objective assessment of the individual's physical condition and health status. Factors to be considered would include the patient's age, gender, general health status, medications, musculoskeletal integrity and functional exercise capacity. Data from graded exercise testing should include peak heart rate attained, measured or estimated maximal oxygen uptake, occurrence of ischaemic ST segment displacement, arrhythmias and inappropriate blood pressure response.

For the cardiac patient, the initial training load is lower and the rate of progression slower than for a healthy adult. Patients who have had a myocardial infarction have suffered damage to the myocardium and while this is healing (first 8 weeks) the object of exercise is maintenance of cardio-vascular fitness rather than increasing conditioning. Following this period of time, exercise intensity can be increased to promote a training effect.

Following coronary artery bypass graft surgery, however, patients who have not suffered myocardial damage can start conditioning earlier and progress at a more rapid rate. A percentage of surgical patients do suffer some peri- or postoperative ischaemia or infarction which is indicated by elevated cardiac enzymes and electrocardiographic changes. Care should be taken that these patients are not pushed into higher levels of activity too quickly but should follow a more gradual programme similar to patients who have had a myocardial infarction.

Exercise dose is a combination of intensity, frequency and duration of activity. It should be sufficient to elicit a conditioning effect but not enough to provoke complications. Though aimed at enhancing cardiovascular fitness it should also include exercise for muscular strength, endurance and flexibility. This may need to be personally tailored to suit the individual's vocation and recreational pursuits. Principles and information provided may be basically the same for many patients but the small variations that consider each patient's preferences make the programme individualized, increasing compliance and effectiveness. The interrelationship between frequency, intensity and duration allows a desirable limitation in one factor to be compensated for by adjustment of the others.

Intensity

The most important component of an exercise prescription is intensity. It is best expressed as a percentage of functional or aerobic capacity. Several physiological and biochemical adaptations, associated with improvement in oxygen transport capacity, occur in response to training at intensities between 57 and 78% of maximal oxygen uptake.[11] This is therefore considered the optimum training intensity. For most individuals following myocardial infarction, however, the threshold intensity for exercise conditioning probably falls between 40 and 60% of maximal oxygen uptake, depending upon the pretraining work capacity and habitual physical activity.[12]

Patients can be taught to monitor intensity of exercise using one, or a combination, of several methods. The simplest and most frequently used of these are based on *training heart rate, rates of perceived exertion and metabolic equivalents (MET)*.

Training heart rate. The most common method of establishing an exercise intensity is based on heart rate. As there is a linear relationship between heart rate and oxygen uptake during dynamic exercise, heart rate may be used as an index of oxygen uptake.[13] The target training zone of 57–78% maximal oxygen uptake corresponds approximately to 70–85% of symptom-limited maximal heart rate. This relationship exists regardless of age, gender, body weight or fatness, mode of exercise or medical therapy. When

TABLE 8.2
Scales of Perceived Exertion

Rate of perceived exertion	New rating scale
6	
7 Very, very light	0 Nothing at all
8	0.5 Very, very weak
9 Very light	1 Very weak
10	2 Weak
11 Fairly light	3 Moderate
12	4 Somewhat strong
13 Somewhat hard	5 Strong
14	6
15 Hard	7 Very strong
16	8
17 Very hard	9
18	10 Very, very strong
19 Very, very hard	– Maximal
20	

measured maximum heart rate is not available, the age-predicted maximum heart rate may be substituted (maximum heart rate = 220−age). Care should be taken when using this formula as it does not allow for individual variations or the effects that some medications have on heart rate. These limitations render it suitable for low-risk patients only. The training heart rate range is calculated simply by computing 70–85% of the measured or calculated maximum heart rate.

Another method commonly used is the heart rate reserve method of Karvonen[14] where:

Training heart rate =
[(maximum heart rate − resting heart rate) × 60–80%] + resting heart rate.

This method is particularly advantageous in the early postoperative coronary artery bypass graft patients among whom resting heart rate is frequently higher than 70% of maximum heart rate.[8]

The advantages of using heart rate as an index of training intensity include its simplicity and ease of transfer. Training intensities set in the gymnasium or supervised programme can be applied to various new exercise and recreational activities. It also has a built-in progression. As patients' functional capacity improves they will be able to do more work before achieving their training heart rate.[11]

Rate of perceived exertion. Another simple and transferable method of quantifying exercise intensity is Rate of Perceived Exertion (RPE). RPE is a scale developed by Borg[15] consisting of 15 grades of intensity 6–20. Some workers are now using a revised ratio scale, shown in Table 8.2.

In the early stages of cardiac rehabilitation, intensity in the 12–13 rating (somewhat hard) usually corresponds to the upper training heart rate. In later stages ratings of 13–15 correspond with training heart rates of 70–85% maximum heart rate. Anaerobic threshold is generally reached at an RPE of 13.5 for the cardiac patient. These values are valid regardless of peak heart rate and medications.

RPE is a reliable indicator of the intensity of effort. Patients trained in the use of this method can translate its application across a wide variety of exercise modes and daily activities. It may also be a valuable indicator of how the patient is adapting to training.[16]

MET method. Exercise and activity can also be prescribed using the metabolic equivalent or MET method. A large number of training, recreational and occupational activities have been defined in terms of caloric expenditure per minute or by oxygen uptake and expressed on a relative basis as metabolic equivalents (METs) (1 MET = 3.5 ml of oxygen consumed/kg/min). The major advantages of this method are that it remains accurate despite alteration of medical therapy and that METs are available for a large number and variety of activities. Tables listing MET values are available in many cardiac rehabilitation and exercise physiology textbooks.[2,7]

With this method, exercise is prescribed by determining a percentage of the individual's functional capacity and selecting activities that fall within that range. Generally 60–75% of maximal METs achieved on exercise testing is considered an appropriate training intensity. For physical activities such as walking, cycling and stair climbing, the MET level is directly related to the speed of movement and measurable resistance.

There are problems with the use of this method as it does not allow for other variables such as emotional stress, cognitive demands and environmental influences (temperature and humidity) which may alter the cardiac demands of an activity. Unlike the other methods described this method has no built-in progression of training intensity. Therefore, as patients adapt to conditioning, periodic evaluation may be necessary to update the exercise prescription.

Duration

Guidelines for exercise testing and prescription produced by the American College of Sports Medicine[12] suggest that the conditioning phase of an exercise session should be 15–60 minutes in duration. For most patients a suitable duration for conditioning is 20–40 minutes. This does not include the time spent warming up and cooling down.

The conditioning effects resulting from an exercise programme are related to the total energy expenditure. This is the product of intensity and duration of exercise. High-intensity, short-duration programmes are usually unsuitable for cardiac patients as they carry a greater risk of eliciting cardiac symptoms and musculoskeletal injury.

Warm-up should be 10 minutes in duration and consist of a locomotor activity and flexibility exercises. Usually the best warm-up activity is the same activity as the conditioning activity but performed at a lower level. Appropriate warm-up will allow gradual physiological adaptation in preparation for the exercise to follow. Intensity should be sufficient to increase heart rate to within 20 beats of the target heart rate. This minimizes the risk of cardiovascular and musculoskeletal complication.[13]

A 5–10 minute cool-down should include low-level exercise or walking to enhance recovery from the conditioning phase. It permits rapid re-adjustment of the circulation to near resting levels whilst facilitating rapid removal of the post-exercise metabolic wastes. Neglecting to cool-down properly can allow a transient decrease in venous return which may result in reduced coronary blood flow while demands are still high. This increases the chances of ischaemia and/or arrhythmias. Haskell[17] reports that of 61 cardiovascular complications occurring in cardiac patients during exercise 78% occurred during either the warm-up or cool-down phases.

Frequency

The most desirable frequency depends on the intensity and duration of the exercise sessions. It may vary from several sessions per day to three weekly sessions. In the early phases of rehabilitation when patients have low functional capacity, frequent short sessions of low intensity are most suitable. As fitness improves duration and intensity of sessions may be increased and frequency decreased. Three to five sessions per week with a 30-minute conditioning component are commonly prescribed in the later phases of rehabilitation.

Mode

Mode of exercise should be selected carefully as there are many factors to consider. Endurance activities are the most suitable for increasing and maintaining functional capacity. These would include any activity which entails the use of large muscle groups in a rhythmical, repetitive fashion over a prolonged duration of time and is therefore aerobic in nature.

Walking should be the primary mode of inpatient exercise for most patients as this will most likely be their mode of exercise post discharge. Its advantages are its simplicity and lack of requirement for special skills or equipment. It is also the most functional of exercise modes. Patients who have stairs at home should also have stair climbing included in their inpatient activity programme.

Some patients will have access to exercise bikes at home and for these patients stationary cycling may be commenced as inpatients. Exercise bikes are useful when the weather is inclement, either wet, cold or too hot and for patients who are very overweight or have some other physical problem limiting their ability to walk. Disadvantages with stationary cycling include the monotony of being stationary during exercise and the discomfort some patients experience from the seat. Another limitation is that many exercise bikes do not have reproducible intensity controls making it difficulty to provide consistent or progressive intensity between exercise sessions. In these cases it may be of assistance to use RPE to set the intensity of exercise.

Walking and cycling continue to be suitable and commonly prescribed modes of exercise into later phases of cardiac rehabilitation. Other suitable activities include swimming, jogging, some other sports and dancing.

The mode of exercise may be performed in either a continuous or discontinuous (interval conditioning) manner. Interval training is very useful for extremely deconditioned patients as it produces less fatigue and is therefore better tolerated than continuous exercise. It may also be a useful alternative for patients with musculoskeletal limitations or other medical conditions which reduce tolerance to sustained exercise. In most instances regimes of 2-minutes exercise, 1-minute rest or 5-minutes exercise, 2-minutes rest are suitable.

As many of the activities of daily living involve combinations of static and dynamic exercise using both the upper and lower limbs and training effects tend to be activity-specific,[13] it is important to include a component of upper limb exercise in a comprehensive exercise prescription. Although traditionally arm exercise has been viewed with caution for patients with cardiac disorders recent studies indicate the safety and effectiveness of arm exercise for these patients.[18] Ideally, arm exercise should be prescribed on the basis of an exercise test performed using the arms, although in most cases this is often not practical. Maximal heart rate achieved during arm exercise is generally lower than that achieved during leg exercise. Franklin *et al.*[11] suggest that a power output approximating 50% of that used for leg training is appropriate for arm training.

TROUBLE SHOOTING

When devising an exercise programme for cardiac patients, the therapist is often faced with a number of issues to consider. Some of these issues are addressed in the following questions and answers.

Q.   A patient was prescribed on β-blockers following his exercise test. Do I have to retest him to prescribe his exercise?
A.   Not necessarily. β-blockers will not change his functional exercise capacity and the MET method of prescription will therefore, still be valid. Training HRs can then be determined by measuring the patient's HR response (on β-blockers) while steady-state exercising at the lower and upper MET limits is calculated.

Q.   A patient's blood pressure (BP) dropped at peak exercise. Is exercise prescribed in the usual way?
A.   Yes. There is no reason to expect submaximal BP response to be abnormal in these patients.

Q. Post-bypass patients frequently have a resting HR higher than 70% of their HR_{max}.
A. Use the HR reserve method of exercise prescription, 50% of HR reserve is a suitable training level for the early post-bypass patient.

Q. How is intensity best prescribed in patients with fixed rate pacemakers?
A. In these patients the RPE or MET method prescriptions must be used. As the heart rate response to exercise may not occur, maximal cardiac output may be limited and careful attention should be paid to onset of symptoms indicative of insufficient output.

REFERENCES

1. Saltin B.B., Blomqvist J.H., Mitchell R.L., *et al.* (1968). Response to submaximal and maximal exercise after bed rest and training. *Circulation*, **38** (Suppl. 7).
2. Wenger N.K. (1979). Early ambulation after myocardial infarction: Rationale, program components and results. In *Rehabilitation of the Coronary Patient* 2nd edn. (Wenger N.K., Hellerstein H.K. eds). New York: John Wiley and Sons, pp. 53–65.
3. Froelicher V.F. (ed.) (1987). *Exercise and the Heart: Clinical Concepts* 2nd Rev. edn. Chicago: Year Book Medical Publishers.
4. Hung J., Goldwater D., Convertino V.A., *et al.* (1983). Mechanisms for decreased exercise capacity after bed rest in normal middle-aged men. *Am. J. Cardiol.*, **51**, 344.
5. Worcester M. (1986). *Cardiac Rehabilitation Programmes in Australian Hospitals.* National Heart Foundation of Australia.
6. WHO Technical Report Series 270: 1964.
7. Pollock M.L., Ward A., Foster C. (1979). Exercise prescription for rehabilitation of the cardiac patient. In *Heart Disease and Rehabilitation* (Pollock M.L., Schmidt D.H., eds.). Boston: Houghton Mifflin Professional Publishers, pp. 413–445.
8. Metier C.P., Pollock M.L., Graves J.E. (1986). Exercise prescription for the coronary artery bypass graft surgery patient. *J. Cardiopul. Rehab.*, **6**, 85.
9. Naughton J. and Hellerstein H.K. (eds.) (1973). *Exercise Testing and Exercise Training in Coronary Heart Disease.* New York: Academic Press.
10. Miller H.S. (1985). Supervised versus nonsupervised exercise rehabilitation of coronary patients. In *Exercise and the Heart* 2nd edn (Wenger N.K., ed.). Philadelphia: F.A. Davis, pp. 193–200.
11. Franklin B.A., Hellerstein H.K., Gordon S., *et al.* (1986). Exercise prescription for the myocardial infarction patient. *J. Cardiopul. Rehab.*, **6**, 62.
12. American College of Sports Medicine (1986). *Guidelines for Exercise Testing and Prescription*, 3rd edn. Philadelphia: Lea and Febiger.
13. Hellerstein H.K., Franklin B.H. (1984). Exercise testing and prescription. In *Rehabilitation of the Coronary Patient*, 2nd edn. (Wenger N.K., Hellerstein H.K., eds.). New York, John Wiley and Sons.
14. Karvonen M., Kentala K., Mustala O. (1957). The effects of training on heart rate: A longitudinal study. *Ann. Med. Exp. Biol.*, **35**, 307.
15. Borg G. (1970). Perceived exertion as an indicator of somatic stress. *Scand. J. Rehab. Med.*, **2**, 92.
16. Borg G.A. (1977). Perceived exertion: a note on history and methods. *Med. Sci. Sports.*, **5**, 90.

17. Haskell W. (1978). Cardiovascular complications during exercise training of cardiac patients. *Circulation*, **57,** 920.
18. Blomqvist C.G. (1985). Upper extremity exercise testing and training. In *Exercise and the Heart* 2nd edn. (Wenger N.K., ed.). Philadelphia: F.A. Davis, pp. 175–184.

Appendix A

Clinical Reasoning: Case Studies

ELIZABETH ELLIS

INTRODUCTION

The process of clinical decision-making is fundamental to responsible professional practice and quality health care. While it is seemingly an innate characteristic of competent clinicians, it is in fact learned and the discrete steps involve very different skills and processes. This section will examine some of the clinical reasoning processes involved in decisions made about clinical intervention. The process has been described in a simplified manner for clarity. In reality, there are a multitude of issues associated with the provision of health care servces which will influence the therapist's effectiveness and the treatment outcome.

The first section of Appendix A focuses on interpretation of clinical findings which is a critical and integral part of the first three stages of the clinical decision-making process as described in Chapter 1 – assessment, analysis and planning. Interpretation of clinical findings is the careful and systematic tying together of pieces of information gathered from a wide variety of sources and interpreting the overall significance of each piece. This first section consists of case presentations as the person appears on the ward or in a clinic. The cases are presented in couplets on the basis of the apparent similarity of their signs and symptoms. Superficially, the paired cases are very similar and, without the additional information provided by a thorough history, physical examination and test results, would be difficult to distinguish. With the additional information, the analysis of each case is very different and consideration of all the information is needed for effective interpretation. In the description of these case examples, if a sign or symptom is omitted, it is to be assumed that it is not present.

The second section of Appendix A examines some of the issues which must be considered during all stages of the decision-making process. Within the case examples, a brief outline is given of information which could be considered in the decision-making process. The typical way that an adult or child may present is described under the assessment although some of the features may vary despite a similar pathophysiology. Background questions have been provided to act as a stimulus for further reading.

Appendix A does not provide detailed information on intervention but rather emphasizes the importance of careful evaluation of all relevant details and the differences in the goals of intervention. Consideration will be given to the importance of planning strategies for intervention aimed at affecting both the underlying problem and reducing the risk of additional problems developing.

INTERPRETATION OF CLINICAL FINDINGS

Reduced Ventilation

Two individuals present similarly with a cough, breathlessness and an inspiratory wheeze.

Case A1: The history reveals previous good health with an episode of sudden onset of coughing which settled eventually to a persistent mild cough. On physical examination there are localized wheezes and reduced air entry on the right between the 4th and 6th rib anteriorly. Chest X-rays show localized collapse of the right middle lobe. At bronchoscopy an inhaled peanut was identified and removed from the right middle lobe.

Analysis of the information gathered would lead to the conclusion that there had been localized airways obstruction by the peanut, causing reduced ventilation and collapse of the right middle lobe. As the cause of the problem has been removed, it is reasonable to assume that the lung should re-inflate with intervention. The goals of physiotherapy intervention, therefore, would be to re-inflate the right middle lobe and clear any mucus which may have collected. The longer term goal would be to prevent a secondary infection.

Case A2: The clinical history indicated that previously this individual had episodes of wheezing at night and on exertion. The individual has previously had a positive exercise test for exercise-induced asthma. On examination, the patient is pale and distressed with widespread inspiratory and expiratory whistles, with reduced air entry generally. The sputum is yellow and the chest X-ray shows slight hyperinflation.

Analysis of the information gathered suggests that the individual has reduced alveolar ventilation secondary to widespread airways narrowing. The airways narrowing may be reversed by drug therapy and removal of any excess secretions. The goals of physiotherapy, therefore, are to reduce the airways obstruction with effective use of inhaled drugs and sputum removal. The long-term goal would be to reduce the incidence of future episodes of asthma.

Mucocilary Clearance

The two people in this section present with a productive cough and crackles on auscultation.

Case B1: Detailed history revealed that this person had an illness with an acute onset, characterized by a high temperature and general malaise. Physical assessment indicated that he had been otherwise well and had no other signs other than the coarse crackles heard over the lingular segment of the left lung. Chest X-ray indicated that there is a bronchopneumonia in the lingular segment and sputum cultures showed positive bacterial infection.

Analysis of this information indicates that the patient has an acute infection of the bronchus and surrounding lung tissue which is causing excessive secretions in the bronchus of the lingular segment of the lung. Intervention should aim to remove the localized secretions from a lingular bronchus using techniques for sputum removal which will achieve this without causing distress (see Chapter 6).

Case B2: This person had a longstanding history of cough with sputum since childhood, the amount varying with the clinical condition of the individual. On auscultation, medium intensity crackles were heard all over the chest wall, more intensely over the lower lobes. Chest X-ray showed no local lesion. However, there were signs of fibrosis in the lower lobes.

There are excessive secretions throughout both lung fields and the lower lobes appear to be more severely affected than the upper or middle lobes. The condition appears to be longstanding and chronic bronchiectatic changes to the airways should be suspected. The goal of intervention would be to assist with the clearance of the secretions until the patient is returned to a normal state or as best as can be expected with chronic bronchiectatic disease. It would be important to ensure that the individual was able to establish independent on-going treatment in order to remain well.

Exercise Tolerance

The following two individuals both have a reduced exercise tolerance due to breathlessness.

Case C1: On questioning, this person describes marked breathlessness on exertion which resolves spontaneously about twenty minutes after stopping exercise. Following a 6-minute submaximal exercise test, there was marked bronchoconstriction as evidenced by a significant drop in expiratory flow rates and expiratory whistles. The bronchoconstriction returns to normal approximately 30 minutes after the exercise period. The person was otherwise well and did not suffer from breathlessness at any other time.

The signs and symptoms indicate that this person probably has a reversible limitation to exercise (exercise-induced asthma) which is likely to be preventable. The goal of intervention would be to reduce the number and severity of episodes of asthma through education about the appropriate use of bronchodilators. In addition, a programme of graded exercise would reduce the ventilatory demand of exercise and thereby the trigger for this form of asthma.

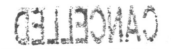

Case C2: This person had a longstanding history of progressive limitation to exercise because of breathlessness. He had chronic airflow limitation which had been treated medically. The lung volumes demonstrated hyperinflation consistent with the disorder. On auscultation, there was reduced air entry with expiratory whistles.

Analysis of the signs and symptoms indicates that this person has a fixed pulmonary limitation to exercise. There would appear to be very little that can be done to reverse the underlying ventilatory impairment.

The goal of intervention would be, therefore, to provide a gradually increasing programme of exercise and breathing control which would enable the individual to perform more work within his ventilatory limits.

Disorders of Cardiac Function

The next two people present similarly with breathlessness and with fine crackles and reduced air entry over both lung bases.

Case D1: From the history, it was found that this person had recently suffered an acute myocardial infarction with considerable damage to the left ventricle. Chest X-rays showed a pattern of pulmonary vascular engorgement and left ventricular enlargement.

This person is suffering from left ventricular failure which is causing pulmonary oedema. Because of the acute nature of the myocardial infarction, the clinical condition is considered quite unstable and care will need to be taken not to increase the load on the left ventricle which would exacerbate the ventricular failure. The goal of intervention would be to try to maintain adequate ventilation without aggravating the ventricular function.

Case D2: This person had a history of marked hypoxaemia secondary to chronic lung disease. On observation and palpation, there was bilateral ankle oedema and raised jugular venous pressure. On auscultation, there was reduced air entry, widespread crackles and inspiratory and expiratory rhonchi. This person was cyanosed peripherally and had clubbing of the fingertips.

Analysis of the information available on this case indicates that there is evidence of right ventricular failure which is probably secondary to the chronic hypoxic effects of the lung disease. The goal of physiotherapy intervention would be to relieve the hypoxaemia by improving ventilation. This may be best achieved by assisting with the removal of secretions.

While each pair of case studies presents examples of people with similar signs and symptoms, thorough analysis of all the information available makes it clear that the goals of intervention for each case should be very different. It is clear that many symptoms, breathlessness in particular, can have a wide variety of clinical causes and are no indication by themselves for the likely direction of intervention.

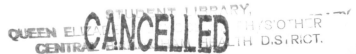

CLINICAL REASONING AND STRATEGY PLANNING IN SPECIFIC CONTEXTS

Childhood Asthma

An 8-year-old boy, who has had asthma since the age of 3 years, is referred to a physiotherapy private practice for assessment and advice. He has been attending school regularly; however, his attendance is interrupted by recurrent infections and he does not usually participate in school sporting activities due to shortness of breath. He has been prescribed a bronchodilator puffer and an inhaled steroid which he uses intermittently when wheezing. On assessment, it is established that he is small for his age and has a slightly pigeon chest. He has widespread expiratory wheeze on auscultation. He otherwise appears a well and happy child. A 24-hour peak flow measurement showed an early morning 'dip' and considerable variation in airflow limitation throughout the day. On a 6-minute exercise test, he dropped by 35% from his resting value of FEV_1.

> There are a number of issues, related to his growth, development and ability to participate in normal activities, which need to be considered for this child. If he is able to exercise without breathlessness then this may allow him to participate more fully with his peers and will also act as a stimulus for more normal growth patterns. It will be important to evaluate the attitudes of the child, the parents and the teachers to medications and to assess how effectively they communicate with each other.

The child appears to have problems of low-grade airway obstruction with recurrent infections and exercise limitation due to responsive airways (exercise-induced asthma). It would also appear that there may be some late reaction, possibly to an allergen, which causes the early morning decrease in airway function. The plan of intervention in the short term would be to try to improve airway function, reduce the exercise-induced asthmatic response and reduce the risk of repeated infections. In the long term, the goal of intervention would include improving exercise tolerance, reducing allergen exposure and reducing any postural and chest wall deformity which may be developing.

> Because there are a number of quite complex goals which potentially affect the child, his family and the school, it will be important to establish the specific goals with the child and parents and form a plan for careful monitoring of the achievement of each of these.

To improve airway function, the technique for using the medications should be assessed and corrected where necessary in order to ensure appropriate distribution of the aerosol droplets within the lungs. Timing of the medications can be discussed with the child and parents to ensure optimal effectiveness, in particular, timing the use of bronchodilator therapy before exercise and demonstrating how this can block exercise-induced asthma. To reduce the effects of respiratory infection, strategies can be worked out to improve his general health, such as those relating to diet and exercise, and early intervention with appropriate medication when an infection develops. As the child's response to exercise improves, an exercise programme could be designed to increase performance and reduce any postural and chest wall deformity. Swimming is often chosen for asthmatic children as an appropriate form of aerobic exercise as it causes the least amount of exercise-induced asthma, involves the upper limbs and trunk, and teaches breathing control. Referral to an allergen testing clinic will be necessary to identify specific allergens to which the child may be sensitive and then strategies can be worked out for reducing the exposure and/or the effect of these.

It may be necessary to follow this child over a period of months in order to assess the effectiveness of the intervention. A diary of symptoms, daily peak expiratory flow measurements, medication use and activities would help the evaluation of progress. Discussion with the teacher and if necessary, the physical educator of the school, on medication use with exercise may be necessary to reinforce the goals.

Background questions to consider:
What are the different triggers to asthma that this boy may have and what are the mechanisms causing the reaction?

What are the possible reasons for his recurrent chest infections?

Under what conditions is his exercise-induced asthma likely to be worse?

What are some of the potential barriers to the effective management of this boy and how would you suggest that they be overcome?

Stable Angina Pectoris

A 35-year-old man has been diagnosed as having stable angina pectoris secondary to coronary artery disease. He has previously been a track and field competitor and is now employed as a factory manager. He is a slightly obese but otherwise fit looking man, who would like to delay surgery for coronary artery grafting until his young family are all at school. He is able to exercise at 65% of his predicted maximal work capacity before he gets angina and signs of ischaemia.

> The factors which may influence this man's outcome include his ability to change aspects of his lifestyle which may be contributing to his coronary artery disease. In addition, there will be work commitments and social pressure which will need to be understood when planning intervention. It may also be important to explore his feelings about himself and his attitude to illness in order to set appropriate goals.

The main problem is the reduced exercise tolerance because of chest pain and breathlessness. In addition, there appears to be significant stress associated with work and family commitments. He has chosen to delay surgery and so in the short term it will be of benefit to try to increase his exercise tolerance within the limits of his angina and to help him lose weight. In the long term it may be possible to reduce other risk factors for coronary artery disease such as training in stress management. In the future, he may need to be prepared for open heart surgery.

A graded exercise programme to increase his whole body endurance will achieve many of these goals and should include exercise at least 3 times per week, working within 75% of his symptom-limited maximum for at least 20 minutes each exercise period. He may well have a preference for the type of exercise that he would like to do considering his previous athletic experience. Brisk walking, swimming, or bicycling at the appropriate intensity could be suitable choices.

To evaluate the effectiveness of the exercise programme, a repeated exercise test after 6–8 weeks would be appropriate and weight monitoring may also enhance compliance by providing feedback about progress. He may also need referral to a dietitian to help achieve the weight loss goal. Referral to an occupational therapist or psychologist may help with stress management and work modification.

Background questions to consider:
What is the difference between stable and unstable angina pectoris?

What are the common risk factors associated with coronary artery disease and which of these are considered reversible?

What are some of the stress management options available and which would you recommend to be suitable for a working lifestyle?

What are some of the potential barriers to compliance with a graded exercise programme and how would you overcome these?

What would be your goals in preparation for surgery?

Chronic Airflow Limitation

A business woman aged 50 years has chronic bronchitis after a past history of heavy smoking. She has had several admissions to hospital with respiratory tract infections in the past two years. She is currently trying to reduce her smoking behaviour. She has three boys at school and college and she is the sole supporting parent. She has a productive cough and uses accessory muscles of respiration at rest. Her lung function tests show that she has moderately severe airways obstruction which is marginally reversible with bronchodilators.

> Her work schedule and social demands will influence both her need for intervention and her ability to comply with intervention. It will be necessary to identify what her specific goals are and select strategies to achieve those goals which will be feasible. In addition, the effects of menopausal changes will need to be considered, particularly the potential effects of any intervention on osteoporosis.

On analysis, her main problem is excessive sputum production. This is interfering with her social commitments and poses an increased risk of recurrent infection. The long-term risk with chronic bronchitis is the development of progressive pulmonary fibrosis which is a very debilitative disease. Part of the plan for intervention is to ensure that she can effectively manage her own respiratory care including sputum removal techniques and the use of medications. In order to reduce her smoking behaviour, the therapist could provide her with appropriate anti-smoking literature and a range of alternative behaviours to disrupt smoking habits. These could include relaxation training, stress management and exercise.

The effectiveness of the intervention could be assessed with a treatment diary that recorded her treatment times and the outcome, behavioural changes and incidences of infection. It may be appropriate to refer her to a quit-smoking programme and a dietitian for nutritional advice and calcium intake review.

Background questions to consider:
What are the pathological changes in the airways with chronic bronchitis that increase the risk of infection?

What menopausal changes may alter the rate of progress of the disease?

What effect does smoking have on the lungs and how is it a risk factor for chronic bronchitis?

How could this woman assess her own chest for the location of specific problems at home in order for her own treatments to be as efficient as possible?

Lung Cancer in the Elderly

A 70-year-old man has had an investigative thoracotomy, which revealed an inoperable tumour of the left main bronchus. It has been decided that he will have radiotherapy for the cancer. He was previously living independently in a supportive community. He complains of pain from the incision, however, he is quite mobile in bed although limited by the intercostal catheters and underwater drains. On the left side of the chest, there is reduced expansion of the chest wall and markedly reduced air entry. There are coarse crackles over the left base and his cough is weak and moist. Chest X-ray shows reduced lung volumes, particularly on the left, with collapse of the basal segments of the left lower lobe.

> Among the many issues to consider at this time are the patient's and the therapist's attitude to death and dying and the effect that this may have on motivation in the postoperative period. The patient's understanding of the effects of radiation, and the type of lifestyle to which he may may wish to return should also be considered.

It appears that this man has postoperative collapse of the basal segments of the left lower lobe. This may be contributed to by partial obstruction of the bronchus by the tumour. He is at risk of significant sputum retention because of the loss of lung volume, the partial obstruction of the airway and the pain from the incision.

The short-term goals would be to re-inflate the lung and to remove excess secretions. In the long term restoration of functional capacity may be important if he is to continue to live independently. In order to achieve the short-term goals, careful positioning will help re-inflate the lung and remove excess secretions. Within the limits of his pain, slow deep breaths with inspiratory hold will help open up lung units. In addition, if he can participate comfortably, the forced expiratory technique (FET) and huff coughing will help remove secretions. In order to restore his functional capacity, a programme of early mobilization with a gradual increase in exercise tolerance should be instituted. Considerable care must be taken in this postoperative period because of the severe pain that thorocotomy patients experience and the fact that they often have postural hypotension on sitting or standing upright.

Monitoring of X-ray changes and auscultation will help evaluate the effect of the short-term intervention. A simple measurement of exercise performance such as the 6-minute walk or step test could be used to assess changes in functional capacity.

Background questions to consider:

What are the possible effects of radiation on tumour growth?

What are the side-effects of radiation on the rest of the human body?

What are the effects of chemotherapy?

What are the side-effects of chemotherapy?

What are the effects of surgery on normal mucociliary clearance?

What are the effects of surgery on ventilation?

Multiple Injury After Motor Vehicle Accident

This 25-year-old man has injuries after a motor vehicle accident which include multiple limb fractures and fractured ribs 7 to 10 on the right lateral chest wall. He has been admitted to neurosurgery intensive care because of a head injury and a ruptured diaphragm which necessitates assisted ventilation. His chest X-rays show regional hypoventilation of the dependent portions of the lung. Arterial blood gases show a mild arterial hypoxaemia and a normal carbon dioxide level consistent with this degree of hypoventilation. On auscultation there are crackles and reduced breath sounds on the right below the line of the nipple. Intracranial pressure is 15 cmH_2O and fluctuates 5 cmH_2O. On admission he was semi-conscious, responsive to pain and had a variable response to simple commands. Both pupils were reactive to light. He is now paralysed and sedated.

This young man is at risk of a number of complications. Firstly, if his respiratory function deteriorates he is at risk of secondary brain damage. Because he is immobilized, he is at risk of respiratory, musculosketetal and neurological complications. It may also be that he has some emotional shock from the accident, especially if friends or family were also involved.

From this assessment it is clear that he has right middle lobe collapse and some mucus retention in that region of the lung. The fractured ribs and variable intracranial pressure will act as precautions to intervention.

After a clear explanation to the patient of the plan of intervention and what to expect, the short-term goal will be to reinflate the right lobes and prevent secondary brain damage by maintaining lung function. In addition, to prevent the musculoskeletal complications of immobilization, intervention to maintain joint range and muscle length should be implemented. Long-term planning should aim for complete rehabilitation with or without nocturnal assisted ventilation depending on the extent of the return of diaphragm function.

The effectiveness of intervention could be assessed by chest X-ray, auscultation, intracranial pressure measurement and functional assessment. It would be of value to have this person's body position varied regularly throughout the day avoiding head-down positions which would cause raised intracranial pressure. In addition, early mobilization would help promote not only ventilation, but also joint and muscle integrity and stimulate return of normal consciousness levels.

Background questions to consider:

What are some of the factors involved in the development of secondary brain damage in the acute head injured patient?

What are the complications of prolonged immobilization and bed rest?

What is the role of physiotherapy in the prevention of complications of intubation and mechanical ventilation?

What are the effects of changing body position on lung volumes?

Appendix B

Positioning

JENNIFER ALISON

POSITIONING TO IMPROVE VENTILATION

In the erect posture, the intrapleural pressure gradient is such that the intrapleural pressure is more negative at the apex of the lung (approx. -10 cmH$_2$O) than at the bases (approx. -2.5 cmH$_2$O). This is largely due to the effects of gravity on the lung. The apex of the lung in this situation is regarded as the non-dependent region, and the bases as the dependent region. The greater negative pressure pull on the alveoli in the apical region means that they are relatively more expanded than those in the basal regions. When a person changes posture to left side-lying, for example, the greatest negative pressure pull is still exerted on the non-dependent region (i.e. the uppermost region) which now is the left lateral side of the lungs. This negative pressure pull will provide a passive expansionary force on the alveoli in this region. When areas of the lung are atelectatic the expansionary pull on the non-dependent alveoli can be used to advantage. If the region of atelectasis is positioned so that it is non-dependent, the greater negative intrapleural pressure in the region will apply a passive expansionary force to the underlying alveoli and will aid re-expansion.

The optimal position in which a particular lobe of segment of the lung would experience the greatest effect of 'positioning' would be to place it in the most non-dependent position. This position is the same as the postural drainage position for that lobe. These positions are called 'specific positioning' for that lobe or segment. Sometimes when specific positioning is contra-indicated, for example, where there is extreme shortness of breath, uncontrolled hypertension, excessively raised intracranial pressure, oesophageal surgery, abdominal distension, orthopnoea, or severe cardiac failure, 'non-specific' positioning is used. In such cases the person's position is altered to make the dependent region of the lung as non-dependent as possible, within the limitations of contra-indications, and, in so doing, aid in re-expansion or improve air entry to the region. Such positions include right or left side-lying, prone or semi-recumbent.

POSITIONING FOR POSTURAL DRAINAGE

Postural drainage is a technique by which a particular lobe of the lung is positioned at 90° to the horizontal so that gravity can aid the movement of secretions from peripheral airways towards the central airways, from where they can be expectorated.

Positions for Specific Segments

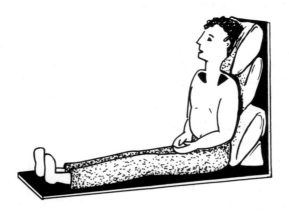

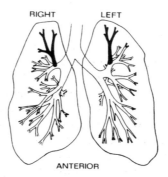

Figure B.1   UPPER LOBE: APICAL SEGMENTS
Postural Drainage Position: *Sitting upright, with slight variations according to the site of the lesion, for example, leaning slightly backwards or forwards. The darkened area represents the lung segment being drained.*

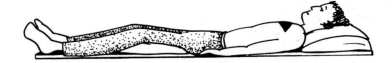

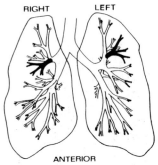

Figure B.2 UPPER LOBE: ANTERIOR SEGMENTS
Postural Drainage Position: *Lying supine with the bed flat. Knees should be comfortably supported with a pillow. Shoulders must not be on the pillow.*

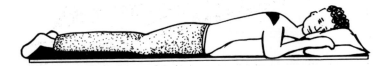

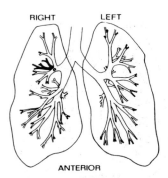

Figure B.3 RIGHT UPPER LOBE: POSTERIOR SEGMENT
Postural Drainage Position: *45° from prone, right (R) side raised by pillows placed comfortably under the R side of trunk and R arm.*

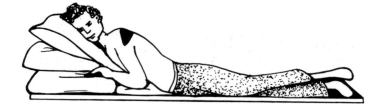

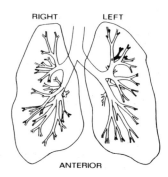

Figure B.4   LEFT UPPER LOBE: POSTERIOR SEGMENT
Postural Drainage Position: *Lying on R side, 45° turned from prone with pillows arranged to lift the shoulders 30 cm.*

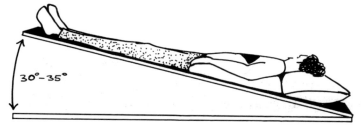

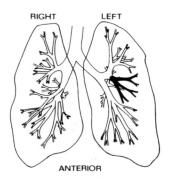

Figure B.5   LEFT UPPER LOBE: LINGULAR SEGMENT (superior and inferior bronchi)
Postural Drainage Position: *Supine, body turned 45° to R and supported by a pillow under left (L) side of back. Foot of bed raised 30–35 cm. R shoulder must not be on pillow. Support under waist if necessary.*

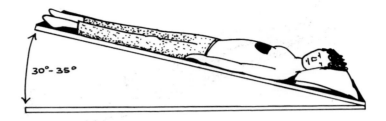

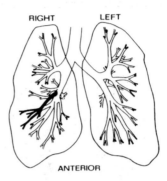

Figure B.6   RIGHT MIDDLE LOBE: LATERAL AND MEDIAL SEGMENTS
Postural Drainage Position: *Supine, body turned 45° to L, that is, R side raised off bed by pillows. Foot of bed raised 30–35 cm. L shoulder must not be on pillow. Support under waist if necessary.*

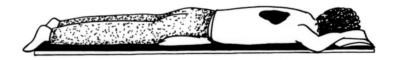

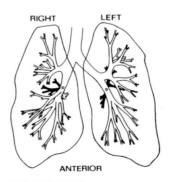

Figure B.7   LOWER LOBES: APICAL SEGMENTS
Postural Drainage Position: *Prone with bed flat and pillow under hips. Shoulders should be relaxed on to bed so that trunk is flat.*

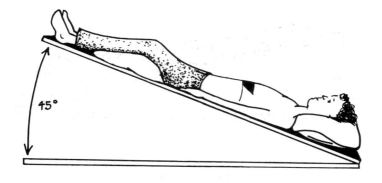

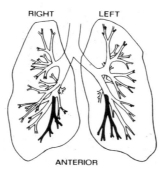

Figure B.8   LOWER LOBES: ANTERIOR BASAL SEGMENTS
Postural Drainage Position: *Supine, foot of bed raised 45 cm. Shoulders must not be on pillow.*

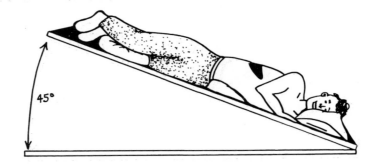

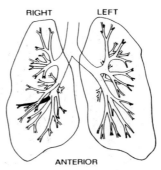

Figure B.9   RIGHT LOWER LOBE: LATERAL BASAL SEGMENT
Postural Drainage Position: *Lying on side with R side uppermost, pillow under waist. Raise foot of bed 45 cm. Support patient with pillow behind trunk if necessary. Shoulder must not be on pillow.*

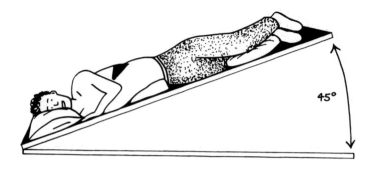

45°

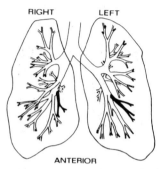

RIGHT LEFT

ANTERIOR

Figure B.10 LOWER LOBES: LEFT LATERAL BASAL AND RIGHT MEDIAL BASAL SEGMENTS
Postural Drainage Position: *Lying with L side uppermost, pillow under waist. Raise foot of bed 45 cm. Support patient with pillow behind trunk if necessary. Shoulder must not be on pillow.*

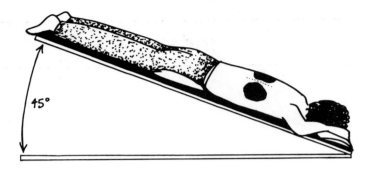

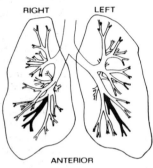

Figure B.11   LOWER LOBES: POSTERIOR BASAL SEGMENTS. Postural Drainage Position: *Prone, with pillow under hips. Raise foot of bed 45 cm. Shoulders should be relaxed into the bed so that trunk is flat.*

Index

Abdomen, 11, 81, 91–5
  gas volume of, 45
  muscles of, 14
  surgery of, 92–5
Abscess:
  pneumothorax and, 73
  radiology and, 65, 78
Accessory muscles:
  asthma and, 96–7
  examination of, 8, 14
  kyphoscoliosis and, 88
Adenosine triphosphate, 131–2
Aerobic metabolism, 132
Airflow meter readings, 34–5
Anaerobic metabolism, 132
Analysis, 2, 80, 82–3, 101–2, 170
  case studies of, 170–9
Angina pectoris, 175–6
Apnoea, 14
  sleep, 14, 88
Arm exercise, 137, 167
Ascites, 92
Assessment, 1–2, 5–23, 170
  case studies of, 170–9
  by function tests, 24–54
  by history, 6–7, 170
  physical, 8–23, 170
Asthma, 96–8
  case studies of, 171, 172, 174–5
  childhood, 174–5
  exercise-induced, 147–8, 171, 172,
    174–5
  mucociliary clearance in, 108
  pulmonary function tests in, 29, 36
Atelectasis (lung collapse):
  examination of, 16–17
  mucociliary clearance and, 115, 121,
    180
  pneumonia and, 91
  post-traumatic, 178–9
  radiography and, 65–70

Auscultation, 19–22
Autogenic drainage, 117–18

Barrel chest, 9, 98
Bedrest, 158
Beta-blockers, 167
Bicycle riding, 136–7, 166–7
Bone(s), 86–8
  examination of, 9–11, 15–16
  fractures of, 178–9
  see also Rib cage
Bradypnoea, 14
Brain, 80, 83
Breath(ing):
  control exercises, 116–17
  dysfunction, 80–102, see also
    individual disorders
  exercise and, 134
  glossopharyngeal, 124
  nervous control of, 80–1, 83–4
  oxygen cost of, 142–3
  patterns, 11–14, 15
  sounds, 19–21
Breathlessness, see Dyspnoea
Bronchitis, chronic, 176–7
Bronchodilator drugs, 123, 174
Bronchophony, 21
Bronchovesicular sound, 20
Bucket handle motion, 11

Cancer:
  of elderly, 177–8
  pneumothorax and, 73
  radiology and, 64, 69, 71–2, 78
Cardiac disorders, see Heart
Chest:
  clapping, 111, 116–17
  configuration, 9–11
  pain, 7, 89, 90
  palpation of, 15–16
  vibration/shaking/compression of,
    113, 116

Chest – (*cont.*)
  wall deformities, 27, 87–8, 140–1
  X-ray, 46, 56–75
Chronic airflow limitation, 26, 98–101
  case study of, 176–7
  exercise and, 138–40
Cilia, 106–7
  dysfunction of, 108–9
  see also Mucociliary clearance
Clapping, chest, 111, 116–17
Clavicles, 10–11
Clubbing, 9, 99
Collapse, *see* Atelectasis
Collateral ventilation, 115, 121
Compensatory strategies, 82
Compliance of lung, 52–4
Compression, 113, 116
Computerized tomography, 76–8
Consolidation, 62–4, 75
Continuous Positive Airway Pressure,
  91, 120
Cor pulmonale, 75, 173
Costal indrawing, 14
Cough, 113
  assessment of, 7
  impairment of, 48
  pneumonia and, 89
Crackles/crepitations, 20–1, 171–2
Creatine phosphokinase, 132
Cyst(s):
  hydatid, 61
  radiology and, 61, 72, 76–8

Decision-making, 1–4, 80, 82–3, 101–2,
  170
  case studies of, 170–9
Diaphragm(atic):
  abdominal surgery and, 92–5
  breathing, 116–17
  breathing patterns and, 11, 14
  chronic airflow limitation and, 100
  fatigue of, 145
  kyphoscoliosis and, 88
  percussion of, 19
  pressures, 93
Diffusing capacity (D_{LCO}), 51–2
Diffusion defects, 142
Dyspnoea (breathlessness), 131
  assessment of, 7, 14
  asthma and, 96–8
  Borg Score of, 150
  case studies of, 172–3
  chronic airflow limitation and, 98,
    101, 140
  fear of, 148–9
  interviewing and, 7

Elastic recoil, 52–4

chronic airflow limitation and, 100,
  101
  work to overcome, 142–3
Electromyogram, 145
Embolism, pulmonary:
  heart failure and, 75
  radiography and, 69
Emphysema:
  pulmonary function tests and, 36, 38
  radiography and, 72
  subcutaneous, 16
Empyemas:
  drainage of, 71
  radiology and, 78
'Energy stealing', 143
Entonox, 124
Environmental factors, 6, 7, 108
Evaluation, 2–3
  of exercise programmes, 149–50
Examination, physical, 8–23, 170
Exercise (activity):
  limitations to, 137–49, 172–3
  mucociliary clearance and, 108, 123–4
  physiology of, 131–4
  psychological benefits of, 149
Exercise programmes, 134–7
  case studies of, 150–4
  compliance with, 149
  evaluation of, 149–50
  in heart disease, 162–8, 176
  muscle, 145–7
  thoracic expansion, 115
Exercise-induced asthma, 147–8, 171,
  172, 174–5

Fibrosis, pulmonary, 89
Finger clubbing, 9, 99
Fissures, pulmonary, 61–2
  collapse and, 67–9
Flow-volume loop, 35–9
Forced expiration technique (FET),
  116–17
Forced expiratory volume in one
  second (FEV_1), 24, 25–7, 31
  airflow meter reading and, 34
  mucociliary clearance and, 111, 121
Forced vital capacity (FVC), 25, 28–9, 31
  mucociliary clearance and, 111, 121
Foreign body, inhaled, 72, 171
Fremitus, 17
Functional capacity:
  functional assessment of, 22–3
  pulmonary function tests of, 24–54
Functional residual capacity (FRC),
  40–5, 46–7

mucociliary clearance and, 120
Funnel chest, 10

Glossopharyngeal breathing, 124
Goblet cells, 105–6
Gravity, mucociliary clearance by, 110, 180
Guillan–Barré syndrome, 84–6

Hamartoma, 72
Heart (disease):
  angina, 175–6
  case studies of, 173, 175–6
  complications of, 160
  failure, 74–5, 173
  output, 134, 135
  rate, 136, 163–4, 167, 168
  rehabilitation in, 158–62
    exercise and, 162–8, 176
  size of, 59
Helium dilution technique, 40–3, 45–6
History, clinical, 6–7, 170
Huffing, 116
Humidification, 122–3
Hydatid cysts, 61
Hyperinflation, 46, 48
  asthma and, 96
  chronic airflow limitation and, 99–101, 139
  reduction of, 46–7
Hyperpnoea, 14
Hyperpnoeic loading, 146
Hyperventilation, 14
Hypoventilation, 83
  abdominal surgery and, 94–5
  kyphoscoliosis and, 88
  pneumonia and, 90
Hypoxaemia, 141–2, 173

Incentive spirometry, 121–2
Inhalation therapy, 98, 101, 123, 174–5
Injuries, multiple, 178–9
Inspiratory capacity (IC), 40, 42–3
Intensive upper body exercise, 146, 147
Interdependence, phenomenon of, 115, 121
Intermittent positive-pressure breathing, 94, 119–20, 147
Interstitial disease, 27
  pneumothorax and, 73
  radiography and, 65
Intervention, 2, 82–3, 101–2
Interview, patient, 7

Kerley 'B' lines, 74
Kyphoscoliosis, 9, 87–8

Kyphosis, 10

Left ventricular failure, 74–5, 173
Lung volumes, 39–47
  abdominal surgery and, 93–4
  reduction in, see Restrictive lung disease

Magnetic resonance imaging, 78–9
Maximal expiratory pressure ($P_E$max), 48–50
Maximal inspiratory pressure ($P_I$max), 47–50
Maximum expiratory flow ($\dot{V}_E$max), 35–9
Maximum mid-expiratory flow rate ($FEF_{25-75\%}$), 25, 29, 31
Mechanical ventilation:
  functional assessment and, 22–3
  muscle weakness and, 48, 144
Medical records, review of, 6
Mesothelioma, 78
Metabolic equivalents (METs), 165, 167, 168
Mid-axillary line, 10–11
Mid-clavicular line, 10–11
Mid-sternal line, 10–11
Mucociliary clearance, 105–28
  abnormal, 108–9
  case studies in, 124–8, 171–2, 176–7, 178
  drainage techniques for, 110–24
  positioning for, 110, 180–8
Muscles, respiratory, 81, 84–6
  asthma and, 96–7
  chronic airflow limitation and, 100
  examination of, 8, 14, 17–18
  exercise and, 131–4, 142–3
    training and, 134–5, 137, 145–7
  fatigue of, 143–7
  kyphoscoliosis and, 88
  measurement of, 47–50
  oxygen requirements of, 142–3
  paralysis of, 124
  pneumonia and, 90
  spasm of, see Asthma
  wasting of, 8, 18, 148
  weakness of, 26–7, 47–8, 84–6, 143, 144
Muscular dystrophies, 84

Nail beds, 8–9, 98–9
Nasal flaring, 14
Nebulization, 122–3
Nervous system, 80–1, 83–4
Neuromuscular disorders, 84–6

Neuromuscular disorders – (cont.)
pulmonary function tests in, 27, 38,
47–8
Nutrition, exercise and, 148

Observation, 8–15
at interview, 7
Obstructive lung disease, 95–101
breath sounds in, 21
case studies of, 171, 174–5
exercise and, 138–40
pulmonary function tests in, 25–6,
28, 30, 46
treatment of, 46–7
see also Asthma; Chronic airflow
limitation
Oedema, pulmonary:
heart failure and, 74–5
radiography and, 62, 74–5
Oral high-frequency oscillation, 112
Oxygen cost of breathing, 142–3
Oxygen transfer, abnormalities of,
141–2

Pacemakers, 168
Pain relief, 124
Palpation, 15–18
Panting, 115
Peak expiratory flow rate (PEFR), 32–4,
39
Pectoriloquy, whispered, 21–2
Pectus carinatum, 9
Pectus excavatum, 10
Perceived exertion, rate of, 164–5
Percussion, 18–19
mucociliary clearance by, 110–12
Periodic Continuous Positive Airway
Pressure, 91, 120–1
Periodic ventilation, 14
Physical examination, 8–23, 170
Pigeon chest, 9
Planning, 2, 82–3, 101–2, 170
case studies of, 170–9
Pleural cavity, 86
air in, see Pneumothorax
effusion, 86
percussion and, 19
radiology and, 70–1, 75, 78
vital capacity and, 27
friction rub, 17
mesothelioma, 78
pressure changes, 52–3
Pneumonia, 89–91
examination of, 17, 19
radiography and, 62–4
Pneumothorax:
examination of, 16, 17

radiography and, 72–4
Pollutants, exposure to, 6, 7, 108
Positioning, 110, 180–8
Positive Expiratory Pressure (PEP), 91,
118–19
Postural drainage, 181–8
Psychological aspects of exercise, 148–9
Pulmonary function tests, 24–54
Pump handle motion, 11
Purse-lipped breathing, 14, 15

Radiography, 56–76
lung volume estimation by, 46
Râles, 20–1
Recommendations, 3
Residual volume (RV), 39–43, 46–7
Resistive loading, 146
Respiratory control centre, 80–1, 83–4
Respiratory muscles, see Muscles
Restrictive lung disease:
exercise and, 140–1
pulmonary function tests in, 27, 28,
38, 46
Rhonchi, 21
Rib(s), 10–11, 15–16
cage, 81, 87–8, 133
fractures of, 178–9
Right ventricular failure, 75, 173

Scapular line, 10–11
Secretions, see Mucociliary clearance
Shaking, chest, 113, 116
Single leg endurance training, 137
Six-minute walk test, 23, 149–50
Skin colour, 8–9, 98–9
Sleep:
apnoea, 14, 88
mucociliary clearance and, 108
Smoking, 176–7
history of, 6, 7
Sounds:
breath, 19–21
vocal, 21–2
Spinal deformity, 9, 87–8
Spirometry, 3, 24–32
incentive, 121–2
Sputum:
assessment of, 7
clearance of, 108–24, see also
Mucociliary clearance
pneumonia and, 89
production of, 106–7
Static compliance, 53
Sternum, 10–11
Subcutaneous emphysema, 16
Submucosal glands, 106

Surgery:
  history of, 6
  upper abdominal, 92–5

Tachypnoea, 14
Tension pneumothorax, 74
Thorax (thoracic), 81
  bony configuration of, 9–11, 86–8
  expansion exercises, 115
  ventilatory dysfunction and, 86–91
Total body plethysmography, 43–6
Total lung capacity (TLC), 39–40, 46
Trachea, palpation of, 16–17
Training, see Exercise programmes
Transdiaphragmatic pressures, 93
Transfer factor (D_{LCO}), 51–2
Tuberculoma, 72
Tuberculosis, 61, 64, 69
Twelve-minute walk test, 149–50

Ultrasonic nebulizers, 123

Ventilation/perfusion inequality, 91,
    100, 141–2
Ventilatory dysfunction, 80–102, see also
    individual disorders
Vertebral line, 10–11
Vesicular sound, 20
Vibration, chest, 113
Vital capacity (VC), 25, 27–9, 31, 40,
    42–3
  exercise and, 133–4
Vocal sounds, 21–2

Wheezing, 21
  asthma and, 96, 171
Whispered pectoriloquy, 21–2
Whistles, 21

X-ray, chest, 56–75
  lung volume estimation by, 46